You Are What You Eat

Subtitle: Food and Nutrition For Health And Longevity

By Yingxiong Feng

While every precaution has been taken in the preparation of this book, the publisher assumes no responsibility for errors or omissions, or for damages resulting from the use of the information contained herein.

YOU ARE WHAT YOU EAT

First edition. March 24, 2024.

Copyright © 2024 yingxiong feng.

ISBN: 979-8224674701

Written by yingxiong feng.

About The Author:

The author is a TCM doctor, teacher and Buddhist practitioner. He has published 20 books in Buddhism, culture and health.

Praised by many as "The best TCM doctor in New York Chinatown", "Loved by all his patients", "Patients' last hope".

Table of Contents

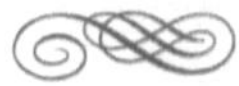

CHAPTER 1

Introduction to TCM Herbal Nutrition

Chapter 2

Nutrition From Foods and Drinks

Chapter 3

Diet and Health for the Elderly

Chapter 4

Dietary Management of Common Diseases in the Elderly

Chapter 5

Common Foods and Their Functions in TCM Terms

Chapter 1
Introduction to TCM herbal Nutrition

Under the guidance of Traditional Chinese Medicine (TCM) theory, our daily food is not only used to satisfy hunger and maintain health, but it also plays a role in preventing and treating diseases, as well as promoting body recovery and delaying aging. Today, we will discuss this issue from the perspective of TCM.

The lifestyle of humans plays an increasingly important role in health and medical care, with the relationship between the two becoming ever closer. As an important part of lifestyle, the study of TCM dietary nutrition includes two major parts: basic theory and daily application. Based on records in historical documents and actual clinical situations, it generally encompasses four aspects: dietary health preservation, dietary treatment, dietary moderation, and dietary dos and don'ts.

The function of dietary consumption is not only reflected in maintaining the normal life activities of the human body, but it also has a nourishing effect, which is different from the viewpoint of modern nutrition science.

From the perspective of Traditional Chinese Medicine, there are approximately one hundred types of daily foods that have significant nourishing effects. These effects include improving hearing, enhancing vision, darkening hair or promoting hair growth, increasing strength, enhancing intelligence, calming the mind, nourishing the skin, beautifying, reducing weight, strengthening teeth, aiding digestion, strengthening muscles, enhancing male virility, assisting in fertility, and prolonging life.

TCM dietary therapy involves using diet to treat or assist in the treatment of diseases. The role of dietary therapy is basically the same as that of medicinal therapy, mainly focusing on supporting the body's vitality and expelling pathogenic factors. The preventive and therapeutic effects of food are also achieved by expelling pathogenic factors, eliminating the causes of disease, supplementing deficiencies, strengthening weaknesses, and adjusting and reconstructing the functions of internal organs to restore the balance of Yin and Yang. The practical application methods are very diverse, making it an important aspect of natural therapy.

The dietary methods advocated by TCM include selecting foods based on the season, local conditions, and individual constitution. It not only emphasizes a balanced diet without bias but also emphasizes moderation in eating. It pays attention to clean foods primarily consisting of grains and meat while also incorporating the consumption of tea and alcohol into the dietary culture to achieve the goal of nurturing the mind and emotions.

The history of dietary culture spanning thousands of years shows that the dietary habits of the Chinese people, as a whole, are based on a foundation of vegetarianism, striving for a balanced mix of vegetarian and non-vegetarian foods, aiming for comprehensive nutrition. The concept of comprehensive nutrition means to diversify the diet as much as possible in terms of content over the long term or regularly, paying attention to the combination of meat and vegetables, main and side dishes, regular meals and snacks, as well as the rational combination of food and drink. It is important not to be biased towards certain types of food, nor to overeat or waste food.

In the field of Traditional Chinese Medicine dietary nutrition, there are specific requirements for dietary taboos in both daily life and clinical practice. These include taboos related to diet and seasonality, constitution, and regional differences; taboos related to food compatibility and interactions with medications; dietary preparation taboos, and dietary taboos during illness.

Traditional Chinese Medicine believes that humans exist between heaven and earth, living within the natural environment as a part of nature. Therefore, there is a close and reciprocal relationship between humans and nature, following the same patterns of movement and change. This interconnectedness between humans and nature is reflected in various aspects of human life, including dietary nutrition.

Since ancient times, various ancient schools of thought aimed at health preservation, longevity, and disease prevention have all used theories of harmonious unity between the human body and the natural world to elucidate the laws of human life, aging, illness, and death. At the same time, they have applied the principles of correspondence between heaven and humanity to formulate various measures for rest, labor, diet, and daily life.

Traditional Chinese Medicine (TCM) theory holds that bodily illness is caused by imbalance between Yin and Yang, so treatment and dietary health maintenance are based on regulating Yin and Yang as the fundamental principle. Regarding dietary dos and don'ts, TCM also starts from the perspective of balancing Yin and Yang, suggesting what is favorable when Yin and Yang are in harmony and what is unfavorable when they are not.

The history of TCM demonstrates that food and medicine share the same origin, both being natural products. They have similar properties in terms of form, color, qi or energy, taste, and texture. Therefore, it is very common in TCM to use food alone, medicine alone, or a combination of food and medicine for nutritional health maintenance, treatment, and recovery.

As food and medicine share the same origin and principles, they have an inseparable relationship. Among numerous herbal and formula classics, examples of using food as medicine can be easily found. For instance, using black chicken, mutton, donkey-hide gelatin, pigskin, bird eggs, green onions, ginger, and dates to nourish Yin and Yang, replenish Qi and blood, or regulate gastric Qi, thereby achieving the effects of preventing and treating diseases. Moreover, from a large number of ancient recipes, cookbooks, and tea books, it is also not difficult to find many medicinal ingredients such as goji berries, Chinese yam, astragalus, poria, cloves, cardamom, and cinnamon, which enhance the health benefits of food and prevent diseases.

In modern society, not only high-protein, high-fat, and high-sugar diets have led to cardiovascular and cerebrovascular diseases, cancer, diabetes, and suboptimal health, but also low intake of vitamins, minerals, and dietary fiber has caused many modern civilization-related diseases. This situation has attracted the attention of many knowledgeable individuals.

As people's lives become more stable and material wealth increases, food becomes more refined, which ironically leads to a deficiency in functional nutrition. This is because many nutrients are concentrated in the husks and embryos of grains and fruits. For example, brown rice is rich in nutrients but has a poor taste. After being processed into white rice, vitamins, trace elements, and dietary fiber are almost entirely lost.

The "Huangdi Neijing" was approximately compiled during the Warring States period, about three thousand years ago, and holds a significant position in the history of Traditional Chinese Medicine development. The "Huangdi Neijing" not only laid the theoretical foundation of TCM but also provided systematic discussions on dietary health preservation and dietary treatment, establishing clear principles and implementation methods.

The "Shennong Ben Cao Jing (The Book of Herbs By Shenong)" is the earliest pharmacological work in TCM. It contains many dietary therapy foods such as dates, goji berries, red beans, and longan flesh, with certain discussions on the efficacy, indications, usage, and administration methods of these dietary therapy foods.

In 1331, Hushi Hui, a Mongolian physician of the Yuan Dynasty, authored the "Yinshan Zhengyao (Important Things About Food And Eating)," which is the first well-known nutritional science monograph. It inherited the tradition of integrating food, nutrition, and medicine, paying attention to the health and medical effects of each food simultaneously. The book mainly contains health foods, and the author provides detailed descriptions of the preparation methods and cooking techniques for various foods. It also lists dietary taboos during pregnancy and restrictions on alcohol consumption.

The types of foods commonly consumed in daily life, whether they are cereals, legumes, grains, fruits and their dried counterparts, or various vegetables, can all be selected for dietary therapy and medicinal diets.

Ingredients such as sugar, alcohol, oil, salt, soy sauce, and vinegar, commonly used in daily life, are all components of medicinal diets. Especially alcoholic beverages are indispensable ingredients in preparing medicinal diets. Various aromatic spices used in medicinal diets not only enhance the flavor but also improve the efficacy of the final product. Therefore, they are highly appreciated by people.

The theory of food properties is the result of previous generations summarizing the experiences of the health and medical effects of food through long-term life and clinical practice.

From the experiential perspective of food in both daily life and clinical applications, foods with a cold or cool nature are often considered Yin in nature, possessing properties of nourishing Yin, clearing heat, relieving fire, cooling blood, and detoxifying. On the other hand, foods with warm or hot properties are considered Yang in nature, with effects such as warming the meridians, boosting Yang, promoting blood circulation, dredging meridians, and dispelling cold.

The five primary tastes of food—sour, bitter, sweet, spicy, and salty—have effects that align with those of medicinal substances. Sourness has an astringent effect, bitterness can lower and drain, sweetness can nourish and replenish, spiciness can disperse, and saltiness can soften and solidify.

Therefore, for everyone, understanding the nutritional characteristics and health benefits of commonly used foods and medicines, learning self-care practices, and promoting health and longevity are necessary and meaningful endeavors.

Chapter 2
Nutrition From Foods and Drinks

Nutrition from diet is the foundation for human survival. When food enters the body, it is absorbed by the stomach, transformed by the spleen, and then distributed throughout the body, becoming the essence of grains and water that nourishes the body.

Dietary supplementation should be based on the individual's constitution. Individuals with a pale complexion, fear of cold, preference for warmth, fatigue in the limbs, frequent clear urination, occasional loose stools, pale lips, spontaneous sweating, weak pulse, and pale tongue with swelling may benefit from supplementation. When these individuals fall ill, they may easily experience symptoms of cold, such as aversion to cold, fatigue, cold limbs, intermittent abdominal pain with a preference for warmth and pressure, facial and limb swelling with difficult urination, cold and painful lower back with clear diarrhea, impotence or spermatorrhea, cold uterus leading to infertility, chest and back pain, coughing, and palpitations, or nocturia and urinary incontinence.

Warming the Yang, supplementing the spleen and kidney, is crucial for individuals with Yang deficiency. Among the five viscera, the kidney is the root of the body's Yang Qi, and the spleen is the source of Yang Qi transformation, thus requiring particular emphasis on supplementation.

Traditional Chinese Medicine believes that Yang deficiency is a further development of Qi deficiency. Therefore, individuals with insufficient Yang Qi often exhibit poor mood and are prone to sadness. It is necessary to strengthen mental adjustment and be adept at regulating one's emotions to alleviate sorrow, prevent fear, control joy, anger, and eliminate the adverse effects of negative emotions.

Individuals with Yang deficiency should consume more foods with tonifying Yang effects, such as mutton, dog meat, deer meat, and chicken. According to the principle of nourishing Yang in spring and summer, in the summer, one can consume mutton and Aconite soup to supplement Yang, in conjunction with the peak of Yang in nature, to strengthen the body's Yang.

Food is diverse and has various functions. Nutrient-rich foods generally have different effects, such as replenishing Qi, assisting Yang, nourishing Yin, nourishing blood, generating fluids, and replenishing essence. Most grains, fruits, vegetables, and some poultry, eggs, meat, and dairy products all have tonifying effects.

Foods with purgative properties generally have various effects such as releasing the exterior, dispersing heat, opening orifices, expelling filth, clearing heat, draining fire, drying dampness, promoting diuresis, eliminating phlegm, dispelling wind and dampness, promoting bowel movements, detoxifying, promoting Qi circulation, dispersing wind, promoting blood circulation, cooling blood, and so on.

The preventive role of food in diseases is increasingly being emphasized by the medical community. Scientists have discovered that many foods can prevent various diseases. For example, bitter melon, asparagus, and purslane have been found to have anti-cancer effects.

For instance, pumpkin seeds are rich in zinc, which has excellent medicinal effects in preventing and improving prostate diseases in men.

For instance, garlic is a health-promoting food that benefits the spleen, detoxifies, and nurtures health. Consuming it regularly can invigorate the spleen and stomach, aid digestion, cleanse the intestines, detoxify, and strengthen the body. It is suitable for individuals with weak stomachs, those who overeat greasy foods, as well as for preventing influenza, intestinal infectious diseases, and cancer. It can be consumed with meals. However, excessive raw consumption is not advisable, especially on an empty stomach, and it should not be consumed together with honey.

From the perspective of Traditional Chinese Medicine (TCM) health preservation and anti-aging, among the nourishing foods, those with anti-aging effects mainly focus on tonifying the lungs, spleen, and kidneys. There are many foods in this category, such as lentils, peas, Job's tears, broad beans, polished rice, glutinous rice, millet, rice, barley, black soybeans, buckwheat, soybeans, wheat, walnuts, dates, chestnuts, longan, lychee, lotus seeds, Chinese yam, lotus root, coix seeds, mulberries, hawthorn, ume (Japanese plum), peanuts, lilies, gingko nuts, almonds, water chestnuts, pears, monk fruit, olives, black sesame seeds, goji berries, ginger, coriander, radish, taro, winter melon, garlic, watermelon, apples, lotus leaves, jujube seeds, white sugar, honey, orange peel, mushrooms, tremella mushrooms, wood ear mushrooms, perilla leaves, tea leaves, Chinese toon, crown daisy, papaya, leek seeds, pumpkin, seaweed, kelp, seaweed, razor clams, sea cucumbers, pigskin, milk, quail eggs, pork liver, beef, deer meat, deer fetus, deer antler, chicken, duck, carp, crucian carp, eel, oysters, and so on.

Due to differences in gender, age, physiological conditions, body types, and individual lifestyle habits, there are different requirements for diet. Therefore, the selection of health foods cannot be standardized. The same food may have significant effects on some people, while it may have adverse effects on others. For example, milk is an ideal nutritional food for most people, but some individuals lack lactase in their bodies, leading to discomfort and diarrhea after consumption. Similarly, while some people may experience improved sleep after eating lychee meat, others may experience insomnia due to excessive internal heat.

The continuous changes in climate throughout the four seasons—spring warmth, summer heat, autumn coolness, and winter coldness—affect human physiological functions to a certain extent. Traditional Chinese Medicine believes that adapting diet to the changing seasons helps maintain the balance of Yin and Yang within the body. Generally, in spring, when the weather is warm and everything is thriving, it is advisable to consume light and refreshing foods, such as shepherd's purse porridge. In summer, when the climate is hot and humid, it is recommended to consume sweet and cool foods, such as mung bean soup, lotus leaf porridge, mint soup, watermelon, and winter melon. In autumn, when the weather becomes cool and dry, it is suitable to consume foods that can nourish Yin, such as lotus root porridge. In winter, when it is cold, it is advisable to consume warm foods, such as eight-treasure rice, hotpot lamb, and longan jujube porridge, to nourish the body's essence and Qi. Different geographical environments also have a significant impact on dietary structures. Improper diet may lead to gastrointestinal discomfort, so this factor should also be taken into consideration.

According to Traditional Chinese Medicine theory, the principles to follow in dietary therapy include warming cold conditions, cooling heat conditions, nourishing deficiencies, and clearing excesses.

Food properties refer to four natures: cold, hot, damp, and cool. Food tastes refer to five flavors: sour, bitter, sweet, spicy, and salty.

Generally, cold and cool foods have the effects of clearing heat, dispelling fire, detoxifying, and reducing inflammation. They are suitable for consumption during spring and summer or by individuals with warm-heat conditions. Examples include grains, mung beans, adzuki beans, pears, bananas, and persimmons.

On the other hand, warm and hot foods have the effects of warming the middle, nourishing deficiencies, and dispelling cold. They are suitable for consumption during autumn and winter or by individuals with deficiency-cold conditions. Examples include glutinous rice, meats, crucian carp, and eels.

Different tastes of foods also have different effects. Spicy foods can disperse and moisten, promote blood circulation, strengthen bones and muscles, and enhance the body's resistance. Commonly used foods include scallions, ginger, garlic, peppers, radishes, various types of alcohol, and so on.

Sweet foods can nourish the middle, relieve urgency, and alleviate pain. Commonly used foods include dates, glutinous rice, animal livers, pears, coconuts, tofu, honey, and white sugar.

Sour foods have astringent and consolidating effects. When combined with sweet flavors, they can nourish Yin and moisturize dryness. Commonly used foods include vinegar.

Bitter foods can clear heat, dry dampness, solidify Yin, and when combined with sweet flavors, they can clear heat, promote urination, and detoxify. Examples include bitter melon and tea leaves.

Salty foods have a softening and loosening effect. Examples include seafood, pig kidneys, and pigeon meat.

Lastly, bland foods have a diuretic effect. Examples include barley, white beans, winter melon, lotus roots, peanuts, and eggs.

Foods with health benefits

FOODS THAT CAN ENHANCE or improve hearing: Lotus seeds, Chinese yam, water chestnuts, water spinach, mustard greens, honey.

Foods that enhance or improve vision: Chinese yam, goji berries, water spinach, pig liver, sheep liver, wild duck meat, greenfish, abalone, snails, clams.

Foods that promote hair growth: White sesame, leek seeds, walnut kernels.

Foods that moisturize and beautify hair: Abalone.

Foods that can restore prematurely white hair: Black sesame, walnut kernels, barley.

Foods for male beard growth: Softshell turtle meat.

Beauty and complexion foods: Goji berries, cherries, lychees, black sesame, Chinese yam, pine nuts, milk, lotus stamens.

Foods that strengthen teeth: Sichuan pepper, water spinach, lettuce.

Weight loss foods: Water caltrops, jujubes, walnuts, longan, lotus leaves, oats, green millet.

Foods that improve thin physique and increase weight: Wheat, japonica rice, sour dates, grapes, lotus root, Chinese yam, black sesame, beef.

Foods for enhancing intelligence, brain health, and boosting morale: Japonica rice, buckwheat, walnuts, grapes, pineapple, lychees, longan, jujubes, lilies, Chinese yam, tea, black sesame, black fungus, cuttlefish.

Foods that calm the mind and aid sleep: Lotus seeds, sour dates, lilies, plums, lychees, longan, Chinese yam, quail, oyster meat, yellow croaker.

Foods to enhance mental alertness and reduce fatigue: Tea, buckwheat, walnuts.

Foods for increasing strength and vitality: Buckwheat, barley, mulberries, hazelnuts.

Foods for strengthening bones and physical strength: Chestnuts, sour dates, salt.

Foods that provide endurance: Buckwheat, pine nuts, water caltrops, shiitake mushrooms, grapes.

Foods to stimulate appetite and aid digestion: Spring onion, ginger, garlic, Chinese chives, coriander, black pepper, chili pepper, carrots, radishes.

Foods to tonify kidney yang: Walnut kernels, chestnuts, broad beans, pineapple, cherries, Chinese chives, Sichuan pepper, dog meat, dog penis, mutton, mutton fat, sparrows, deer meat, deer penis, swallow's nest, shrimp, sea cucumber, eel, silkworm pupa.

Foods to enhance fertility and promote safe pregnancy: Lemon, grapes, black-bone chicken, sparrow meat, sparrow brain, eggs, deer bone, carp, perch, sea cucumber.

In addition, "complementary foods" refer to certain foods that, when consumed together, complement each other's nutritional components, thereby promoting dietary balance. Examples include:

Pork liver and spinach both have blood-nourishing properties; one is animal-based while the other is plant-based. Consuming them together can be particularly effective in treating anemia.

Beef is highly nutritious and beneficial for spleen and stomach health, but its rough texture may irritate the stomach mucosa. However, when cooked together with potatoes, it can protect the stomach mucosa.

Tofu is rich in nutrients, and the saponins it contains can promote the excretion of iodine from food, preventing its absorption by the body. Seaweed contains a large amount of iodine, and consuming the two together can enhance nutritional efficiency.

Sheep meat supplements Yang and provides warmth, while ginger dispels cold and maintains warmth. When consumed together, they can expel external pathogens and treat cold abdominal pain.

Chicken meat supplements the spleen and promotes blood production, while millet supports spleen health. Consuming them together facilitates the body's absorption of the nutrients from chicken meat, thereby enhancing blood production function.

Duck meat nourishes Yin and has anti-inflammatory and cough-relieving effects. Yam has stronger Yin-nourishing properties. When eaten together with duck meat, it can eliminate greasiness and enhance lung nourishment more effectively.

Lily bulb has the effects of clearing phlegm and fire, nourishing kidney Qi, and enhancing Qi and blood. Eggs can supplement Yin and blood. When boiled together with an appropriate amount of white sugar, they can nourish Yin, moisten dryness, clear the mind, and calm the spirit, exhibiting unique health benefits.

Fruits generally contain a large amount of potassium and sodium salts, which participate in human metabolism and help maintain body fluids slightly alkaline. Meat contains a large amount of fatty acids, which, after metabolism in the body, can easily make body fluids slightly acidic. Consuming them together can help maintain the acid-base balance of body fluids, promoting overall health.

Foods with therapeutic effects

DISPELLING WIND-COLD type: ginger, green onion, mustard greens, coriander.

Dispelling wind-heat type: tea leaves, fermented black beans, starfruit.

Clearing heat and draining fire type: water bamboo shoots, bracken fern, bitter herbs, bitter melon, preserved eggs, lily bulb, watermelon.

Clearing heat and generating fluids type: sugarcane, tomato, tangerine, lemon, apple, cantaloupe, sweet orange, water chestnut.

Clearing heat and drying dampness type: Chinese toon, buckwheat.

Clearing heat and cooling blood type: lotus root, eggplant, black fungus, water spinach, sunflower seeds, table salt, celery, luffa.

Clearing heat and detoxifying type: mung beans, adzuki beans, peas, bitter gourd, Chinese spinach, shepherd's purse, pumpkin, vegetables.

Clearing heat and relieving sore throat type: olives, monk fruit, water chestnut, egg white.

Clearing heat and relieving summer heat type: watermelon, mung beans, adzuki beans, green tea, coconut juice.

Clearing heat and resolving phlegm type: white radish, winter melon seeds, water chestnut, seaweed, jellyfish, algae, kelp, horned seaweed.

Warming and resolving cold phlegm type: onion, apricot kernel, mustard seed, ginger, Buddha's hand fruit, citrus, osmanthus, tangerine peel.

Stopping cough and relieving asthma type: lily bulb, pear, loquat, peanuts, almonds, gingko nuts, smoked plums, baby bok choy.

Tonifying spleen and stomach type: pumpkin, cabbage, taro, pork stomach, milk, mango, pomelo, papaya, chestnut, jujube, polished rice, glutinous rice, adzuki beans, corn, fig, carrot, Chinese yam, duck meat, vinegar, coriander.

Tonifying spleen and resolving dampness type: Job's tears, fava beans, Chinese toon, radish.

Expelling parasites type: pine nuts, garlic, pumpkin seeds, coconut meat, pomegranate, vinegar, smoked plums.

Promoting digestion type: radish, hawthorn, tea leaves, koji, malt, chicken gizzard, peppermint leaves.

Warming the interior type: chili pepper, black pepper, Sichuan pepper, star anise, fennel seeds, cloves, dried ginger, garlic, green onion, chives, sword bean, osmanthus, lamb, chicken.

Dispelling wind-dampness type: cherries, papaya, Acanthopanax bark, Job's tears, quail, eel, chicken blood.

Diuretic type: corn, adzuki beans, black beans, watermelon, winter melon, bottle gourd, Chinese cabbage, duck meat, carp, crucian carp.

Laxative type: spinach, bamboo shoots, tomatoes, bananas, honey.

Calming the mind type: lotus seeds, lily bulbs, longan flesh, sour jujube seeds, wheat, millet, mushrooms, pig heart, stone fish.

Promoting qi circulation type: yuzu, oranges, tangerine peel, Buddha's hand fruit, kumquat, buckwheat, sorghum rice, sword bean, spinach, white radish, chives, coriander, garlic.

Activating blood circulation type: peach kernel, rapeseed, kudzu root, eggplant, hawthorn, wine, vinegar, earthworm, oyster meat.

Stopping bleeding type: daylily, chestnut, eggplant, black fungus, Indian lettuce, smoked plums, bananas, lettuce, loquat, lotus root, locust flower, pig intestines.

Astringent type: pomegranate, smoked plum, fox nut, sorghum, apple, lotus seed, yellow croaker, catfish.

Liver-calming type: celery, tomato, green tea.

Qi-nourishing type: polished rice, glutinous rice, millet, yellow rice, barley, Chinese yam, Job's tears, indica rice, potato, jujube, carrot, shiitake mushroom, tofu, chicken, goose meat, quail, beef, rabbit meat, crucian carp, grass carp.

Blood-nourishing type: mulberry, lychee, pine nut, black fungus, spinach, carrot, pork, mutton, beef liver, mutton liver, turtle, sea cucumber, grass carp.

Yang-enhancing type: wolfberry leaves, wolfberry seeds, walnut kernel, cowpea, chive, cloves, sword bean, sheep milk, mutton, dog meat, venison, pigeon egg, quail meat, eel, shrimp, razor clam.

Yin-nourishing type: tremella mushroom, black fungus, Chinese cabbage, pear, grape, mulberry, milk, egg yolk, turtle, cuttlefish, pig skin.

100 Herbs That Can Be Consumed As Dietary Supplements

CLOVES, STAR ANISE, sword bean, fennel, thistle, Chinese yam, hawthorn, persicaria, black-striped snake, smoked plum, papaya, hemp seed, butterfly pea, Solomon's seal, licorice, dahurian angelica, ginkgo, white hyacinth bean, white hyacinth bean flower, longan (lychee), cassia seed, lily, mace, cinnamon, schisandra, Buddha's hand, almond (sweet, bitter), seabuckthorn, oyster, fox nut, Sichuan pepper, adzuki bean, donkey-hide gelatin, chicken gizzard, malt, kelp, jujube (Chinese date), monk fruit, erythrina, honeysuckle, wild jujube, fish mint, ginger (fresh, dried), kumquat, goji berry, gardenia, cardamom, fat sea cucumber, poria cocos, citron, lemon balm, peach kernel, mulberry leaf, mulberry, tangerine peel, platycodon, gotu kola, lotus leaf, radish seed, lotus seed, ginger lily, bamboo leaf, soybean sprout, chrysanthemum, endive, yellow mustard seed, polygonatum, perilla seed, kudzu root, black sesame, black pepper, locust bean, locust flower, dandelion, honey, pine nut, sour jujube seed, fresh imperata, fresh phragmites, pit viper, orange peel, mint, coix seed, Chinese chive flower, raspberry, patchouli, ginseng, honeysuckle, rose, pine pollen, pine nut, apocynum, angelica, Ephedra, saffron, tripterygium wilfordii.

Dietary Guidelines

Diverse Foods, Grains as Mainstays

HUMAN DIETS CONSIST of a wide variety of foods. The nutritional composition of various foods varies. Except for breast milk, no single natural food can provide all the nutrients the body needs. A balanced diet must consist of a variety of foods to meet the body's diverse nutritional needs and promote health. Therefore, it is recommended that people consume a wide range of foods.

Grains and Starchy Foods: Grains include rice, wheat, and other cereals, while starchy foods include potatoes, sweet potatoes, cassava, etc. These foods mainly provide carbohydrates, proteins, dietary fiber, and B vitamins.

Animal Foods: Including meat, poultry, fish, dairy, eggs, etc., primarily provide protein, fat, minerals, vitamin A, and B vitamins.

Legumes and Their Products: Including soybeans and other dry beans, primarily provide protein, fat, dietary fiber, minerals, and B vitamins.

Vegetables and Fruits: Including fresh beans, roots, leafy vegetables, fruits, etc., primarily provide dietary fiber, minerals, vitamin C, and carotene.

Pure Caloric Foods: Including animal and plant oils, starch, edible sugar, and alcoholic beverages, primarily provide energy. Plant oils also provide vitamin E and essential fatty acids.

Eat more vegetables, fruits, and tubers

VEGETABLES AND FRUITS are rich in vitamins, minerals, and dietary fiber. There is a wide variety of vegetables, including leaves, stems, flower stalks, solanaceous fruits, fresh beans, and edible algae, with different varieties containing different and sometimes vastly differing nutrient contents. Dark-colored vegetables such as red, yellow, and green ones have higher vitamin content than light-colored vegetables and most fruits. They are major or important sources of carotene, vitamin B2, vitamin C, folate, minerals (calcium, phosphorus, potassium, magnesium, iron), dietary fiber, and natural antioxidants. Kiwifruits, prickly pears, sea buckthorn, and blackcurrants are also rich sources of vitamin C and carotene.

Some fruits may have lower vitamin and trace element content compared to fresh vegetables, but fruits contain richer substances such as glucose, fruit acids (citric acid, malic acid), and pectin. Red and yellow fruits like fresh dates, citrus fruits, persimmons, and apricots are rich sources of vitamin C and carotene.

Tubers are rich in starch, dietary fiber, and a variety of vitamins and minerals. It is encouraged to eat more tubers. A diet rich in vegetables, fruits, and tubers plays a very important role in maintaining cardiovascular health, enhancing disease resistance, reducing the risk of dry eye disease in children, and preventing certain cancers.

Regularly consume dairy products, legumes, or their derivatives

DAIRY PRODUCTS NOT only contain rich high-quality protein and vitamins but also have a high calcium content with high bioavailability, making them an excellent natural source of calcium.

Legumes are rich in high-quality protein, unsaturated fatty acids, calcium, as well as vitamins B1, B2, and niacin.

Regularly consume moderate amounts of fish, poultry, eggs, and lean meat, and limit the intake of fatty meat and animal fats

FISH, POULTRY, EGGS, and lean meat are excellent sources of high-quality protein, fat-soluble vitamins, and minerals. The amino acid composition of animal protein is more suitable for human needs, with a higher content of lysine, which helps supplement the deficiency of lysine in plant protein. Iron in meat is well absorbed, and unsaturated fatty acids found in fish, especially seafood, help lower blood lipids and prevent blood clot formation. Animal liver is extremely rich in vitamin A and also contains high levels of vitamin B12, folic acid, and other nutrients. However, some organs such as the brain and kidneys contain high levels of cholesterol, which is not conducive to preventing cardiovascular diseases.

Fatty meat and animal fats are high-energy and high-fat foods, excessive intake of which often leads to obesity and is a risk factor for certain chronic diseases, so they should be consumed sparingly.

Food intake should be balanced with physical activity to maintain a suitable weight

FOOD INTAKE AND PHYSICAL activity are the two main factors controlling weight. Food provides energy to the body, while physical activity consumes energy. If food intake is excessive and physical activity is insufficient, the surplus energy will be stored in the body as fat, leading to weight gain and eventually obesity. Conversely, inadequate food intake and excessive physical labor or exercise can result in weight loss due to insufficient energy, leading to decreased labor capacity. Therefore, it is important for individuals to maintain a balance between food intake and energy expenditure. Those engaged in mental work or with low levels of physical activity should strengthen exercise and engage in suitable activities such as brisk walking, jogging, swimming, etc. Underweight children should increase food intake and fat consumption to maintain normal growth and development and achieve a suitable weight. Both excessive and insufficient weight are unhealthy and can weaken resistance, making individuals susceptible to certain diseases such as chronic diseases in the elderly or infectious diseases in children. Regular exercise enhances the function of the cardiovascular and respiratory systems, maintains a good physiological state, improves work efficiency, regulates appetite, strengthens bones, and prevents osteoporosis.

Water chestnuts, winter melon, cucumber, yam, bamboo shoots, sweet potatoes, hair seaweed, black fungus, konjac, and other foods are ideal for weight loss.

Eating a light and low-salt diet

EATING A LIGHT AND low-salt diet is beneficial for health, which means avoiding overly greasy and salty foods, excessive intake of animal-based foods, and fried or smoked foods. The World Health Organization recommends a daily salt intake of no more than 6 grams per person. Dietary sources of sodium include not only salt but also high-sodium foods such as soy sauce, pickles, monosodium glutamate (MSG), and processed foods containing sodium. It is advisable to develop a habit of consuming a low-salt diet from a young age.

Limit alcohol consumption

WHEN IT COMES TO ALCOHOL consumption, moderation is key. During holidays, celebrations, and social gatherings, people often indulge in alcohol. However, alcoholic beverages are high in energy and devoid of other nutrients. Excessive alcohol consumption can lead to decreased appetite, reduced food intake, and various nutrient deficiencies. In severe cases, it can even cause alcoholic liver cirrhosis.

Overconsumption of alcohol increases the risk of high blood pressure, stroke, accidents, and violence, posing harm to both individual health and social stability. Binge drinking should be strictly avoided, and if alcohol is consumed, it should be in moderation, with a preference for low-alcohol beverages. Adolescents should refrain from alcohol consumption.

Eat only clean and hygienic food

IT IS IMPORTANT TO eat clean, hygienic, and non-perishable food. When purchasing food, choose items with a good appearance, free from dirt, impurities, discoloration, and odor, and that meet hygiene standards to prevent diseases from entering through the mouth. Pay attention to hygiene conditions during meals, including dining environment, tableware, and the health and hygiene of food providers. Encourage the practice of separate dining in collective dining settings to reduce the risk of disease transmission.

Chapter 3
Diet and Health for the Elderly

The study of health preservation in traditional Chinese medicine inherits the essence of traditional Chinese medicine theory and ancient philosophical thoughts, taking the holistic view of the correspondence between nature and humans and the unity of form and spirit as its starting point. It advocates looking at life and its activities from a comprehensive analysis perspective. The methods of health preservation are based on the fundamental principles of maintaining the mutual integration of activity and rest, balance, and coordination. It advocates cultivating positive energy, emphasizing prevention as the main approach, and highlighting the importance of dialectical thinking. It requires people to conscientiously and correctly apply the knowledge and methods of health preservation and healthcare with perseverance, through self-care and self-treatment, to improve physical fitness and the ability to resist aging and prevent disease, thus achieving the goal of extending life.

The strength of the body's vitality and the length of life depend on the abundance or decline of the original qi; the biochemical process of metabolism is called physiological qi transformation; the phenomenon of life originates from the ascending and descending movement of qi, which all reflect that qi is not only the basic substance of the human body but also the driving force of life.

The life activities of the human body are based on the internal organs, yin and yang, and qi and blood. Only when there is a balance of yin and yang, qi and blood in the organs can the human body be healthy, free from illness, less prone to aging, and life expectancy can be prolonged.

Diet is the source of nutrients for the body and an indispensable condition for maintaining human growth, development, completing various physiological functions, and ensuring the survival of life.

Dietary health preservation is to adjust diet according to the theory of traditional Chinese medicine, pay attention to dietary taboos, and reasonably intake food to promote health and longevity.

The purpose of dietary health preservation is to supplement nutrients reasonably and moderately to nourish essence and qi, and through dietary adjustment, correct the imbalance of yin and yang in the organs, thereby enhancing physical health and resisting aging and prolonging life.

Reasonably arranging the diet to ensure adequate supply of nutrients to the body can make the qi and blood abundant, the functions of the internal organs vigorous, metabolism active, vitality strong, adaptability to changes in nature, and the ability to resist pathogenic factors strong.

According to the characteristics of food qi and flavor, as well as the condition of the body's yin and yang, providing appropriate dietary nutrition is an important measure to prevent illness. For example, consuming animal liver can nourish the liver and prevent night blindness; consuming kelp can supplement iodine and vitamins, as well as prevent thyroid enlargement. Garlic can be used to prevent colds and diarrhea; mung bean soup can be used to prevent heatstroke.

Many foods have anti-aging effects. For example, sesame seeds, mulberries, goji berries, longan fruit, walnuts, royal jelly, yams, human milk, milk, and turtles all contain anti-aging substances and have certain anti-aging and longevity effects. Regularly choosing appropriate foods for consumption is beneficial for health and longevity.

Dietary health preservation must adhere to certain principles. In general, one should not eat excessively or excessively limit food choices, ensuring a balanced and comprehensive nutrition intake. Moderation is key, avoiding overeating or extreme hunger, and maintaining moderate food intake to achieve the desired health effects. Attention should be paid to dietary hygiene to prevent diseases from entering through the mouth. Tailoring dietary nutrition according to different situations and constitutions is also important, adapting to individual needs and circumstances.

Diet should primarily consist of grains, with meat as a supplementary food, supplemented by vegetables and fruits. People must take a balanced approach according to their needs. Only by adjusting the diet in this way can most of the body's nutritional needs be met, which is beneficial to human health.

Grain foods contain carbohydrates and a certain amount of protein; meat contains protein and fat; vegetables and fruits contain rich vitamins and minerals. These foods work together to meet the body's various nutritional needs.

Excessive hunger leads to insufficient nutrient intake, which cannot guarantee adequate nutrition supply. When consumption exceeds replenishment, the body gradually weakens, inevitably affecting health. Conversely, overeating, consuming large amounts of food suddenly, will inevitably increase the burden on the stomach and intestines, causing food to stagnate in the digestive system, leading to delayed digestion and affecting the absorption and distribution of nutrients; the excessive burden on the spleen and stomach function can also lead to damage.

As bedtime approaches and physical activity decreases, it is not advisable to eat too much. Overeating can cause food stagnation, increase the burden on the stomach and intestines, and lead to indigestion, which can affect sleep.

In the long-term practice of human beings, people gradually realize that some animals and plants are harmful to the human body and can cause food poisoning when ingested, such as dolphins and sprouted potatoes, which are toxic to the human body. Ingesting them can affect health and even endanger life. Therefore, in diet, one should be cautious and carefully identify such items.

Dietary regulation also needs to be arranged according to differences in age, constitution, personality, habits, and other aspects, and cannot be generalized. For example, people with excessive gastric acid should eat more alkaline foods appropriately, while those with insufficient gastric acid should choose acidic foods appropriately to ensure the proper acidity and alkalinity of their diet. Overweight individuals often have phlegm-dampness, so their diet should be light, and they should avoid fatty and greasy foods. Lean individuals often have yin deficiency and internal heat, so they should eat more foods that are sweet and moisturizing, while avoiding spicy and dry foods.

As people reach middle age, typically after the age of 40, signs of aging gradually appear in body shape and function, and it is generally considered that after the age of 65 is the elderly period. As one enters old age, organ functions decline, especially in digestion, absorption, metabolism, excretion, and circulation. Without proper adjustments, this will further promote the aging process.

As age increases, the physiological functions of the human body gradually change, and the demands for dietary nutrition also continuously evolve. For instance, the regulatory function of blood vessels on blood pressure decreases in the elderly, leading to increased peripheral vascular resistance and often resulting in elevated blood pressure. Physiological and pathological changes in the coronary arteries reduce myocardial blood flow and oxygen consumption, further affecting heart function. Immune function declines, making the elderly more susceptible to infectious diseases. Additionally, hearing loss, decreased sense of smell, taste impairment, and other changes occur. Therefore, dietary adjustments should be made according to the characteristics of physiological changes to meet the needs of aging, thereby preventing diseases and delaying aging.

Various factors affect the longevity and health of the elderly, with dietary nutrition being a crucial aspect. Inadequate or imbalanced nutrition is a significant cause of various diseases such as diabetes, hypertension, coronary heart disease, hyperlipidemia, gout, and cancer.

Elderly individuals may experience tooth loss or significant wear due to periodontal disease, dental caries, and atrophic changes in teeth, affecting chewing and digestion of food. Therefore, elderly individuals should eat slowly, chewing food thoroughly and swallowing slowly. This eating habit not only promotes the secretion of various digestive juices, making food easier to digest and absorb, but also stabilizes emotions, avoids overeating, and protects the gastrointestinal tract.

Restricting dietary intake in old age is crucial for health and longevity. If individuals continue to consume the same amount of food in old age, resulting in excess calories, it can have adverse effects on health. Overeating can lead to obesity, which in turn can cause various diseases. Research data show that individuals who overeat and are obese are more likely to die from tumors after middle age than those with normal weight.

Fats and sugars in food are common culprits of obesity in old age. Overconsumption of greasy foods can cause digestive problems and gastrointestinal disorders in elderly individuals with weakened digestive function, thereby affecting the normal absorption of nutrients.

A calm and pleasant mood is conducive to digestion. Optimistic emotions and cheerful moods can greatly increase appetite, as described in traditional Chinese medicine, where a smooth and relaxed liver function leads to a healthy stomach and abdomen. Conversely, negative emotions such as anger and resentment can lead to liver dysfunction and depression, restricting the spleen and stomach, affecting appetite, and hindering digestion.

Elderly people should have a regular diet, with smaller, more frequent meals, avoiding hunger and overeating, and eating at regular intervals and in controlled portions. Following the principle of eating well in the morning, having a full meal at noon, and eating less in the evening can be beneficial.

Elderly individuals should pay special attention to ensuring a certain amount of high-quality protein in their daily diet, such as lean meat, milk, eggs, fish, and various soy products. Additionally, they should eat more foods that have cholesterol-lowering effects, such as onions, mushrooms, black fungus, as well as seaweed and nori, which have some effect in preventing atherosclerosis and reducing the risk of cerebrovascular accidents.

The diet of elderly people should be light and low in salt. Excessive salt intake can lead to hypertension and affect heart and kidney function.

Excessive salt consumption can have adverse effects, especially for the elderly and individuals with heart disease, hypertension, kidney disease, cirrhosis, or ascites. Reducing salt intake is beneficial for preventing hypertension, myocardial damage, and cerebrovascular accidents.

Vinegar not only enhances flavor but also increases gastric acid, improves digestion, stimulates appetite, and kills bacteria, making it a health food for the elderly. Regular consumption of vinegar by the elderly can also soften blood vessels, promote sleep, prevent colds, and provide cooling effects in hot weather.

To adapt to the dental condition and decreased digestive function of elderly individuals, food processing should focus on softening and breaking down food. Cooking methods such as boiling, stewing, simmering, and steaming should be preferred over frying or deep-frying. Additionally, attention should be paid to the sensory characteristics of food, including color, aroma, taste, and appearance, to stimulate appetite.

Moderate alcohol consumption can promote blood circulation and have longevity benefits for the elderly, but excessive alcohol consumption has no benefits and can be harmful.

Coffee consumed by elderly individuals should not be too strong. Strong coffee can accelerate heart rate, leading to premature beats, arrhythmia, excessive excitement, insomnia, and thereby affecting rest and energy recovery. It is especially unsuitable to drink coffee at night. Elderly individuals with atherosclerosis, hypertension, or heart disease are best to avoid coffee altogether.

Elderly individuals should consume food at moderate temperatures. Consuming food that is too cold or too hot can damage the mucous membranes of the digestive tract, especially the esophageal mucosa, which can lead to esophageal cancer over time. Overconsumption of raw or cold food can also damage the spleen and stomach. Elderly individuals should also eat foods that are easy to digest, with food being finely chopped and cooked until soft. They should consume foods rich in vitamins.

A moderate intake of dietary fiber can stimulate intestinal peristalsis and effectively prevent constipation in the elderly. Additionally, dietary fiber also has the benefits of preventing and treating hyperlipidemia, gallstones, colon cancer, and reducing blood sugar levels. Therefore, elderly individuals should ensure an adequate intake of dietary fiber, including a certain amount of whole grains, vegetables, and fruits in their daily diet.

After meals, elderly individuals should regularly massage their abdomen from left to right, repeating the motion approximately thirty times. This method is beneficial for promoting abdominal blood circulation, enhancing gastrointestinal digestion function, and is not only beneficial for digestion but also for overall health.

After eating, oral hygiene should also be emphasized. Food residues are prone to accumulate in the oral cavity after meals, which, if not promptly removed, can lead to bad breath, dental caries, and periodontal disease. Regular mouth rinsing helps maintain oral cleanliness, strengthen teeth, and prevent diseases such as bad breath and dental caries.

It is even more effective to take a walk while massaging the abdomen after meals. Engaging in physical activity after eating helps promote gastrointestinal motility, enhance digestion and absorption, with walking being the best form of activity.

Controlling smoking, maintaining a regular schedule, ensuring adequate sleep, and engaging in moderate entertainment and cultural activities are also essential for maintaining a cheerful mood and abundant energy, which are necessary for ensuring elderly individuals' reasonable nutrition.

Using diet therapy to resist aging and prevent decline

ELDERLY INDIVIDUALS often experience varying degrees of memory decline. Studies have found that foods rich in lecithin, phosphatidylserine, and glutamate can enhance brain activity, delay brain aging, and prevent decline. Foods rich in lecithin include egg yolk, soybeans, honey, chocolate, and others, which are beneficial for brain health.

Due to decreased endocrine function and reduced secretion of sex hormones in elderly individuals, the skin may become dry, wrinkled, and develop pigmentation and spots. However, certain foods can benefit the skin, keeping it smooth and moist. Foods with such effects include lotus seeds, longan fruit, lily bulbs, walnuts, sesame seeds, vegetable oils, and various fruits.

Alzheimer's disease is a common condition among the elderly, characterized by forgetfulness, irritability, and apathy, often negatively impacting happiness in later years. Research by Japanese scientists suggests that consuming egg yolks together with soybeans can help prevent Alzheimer's disease.

Throughout history, traditional medical practitioners have not only discovered many longevity-promoting health foods but also created effective anti-aging formulations. Utilizing these medicines to delay aging and promote fitness is a method known as medicinal diet therapy.

The kidneys are the foundation of innate essence, the root of life, and the source of both prenatal and postnatal essence and energy. When kidney qi is abundant, the body's metabolic capacity is strong, and the aging process is slowed down. Therefore, the effectiveness of longevity-promoting herbal formulations often focuses on nurturing both innate and acquired essence, with a key emphasis on protecting the spleen and kidneys. Other methods such as promoting qi circulation, activating blood circulation, clearing heat, and eliminating dampness are also used to strengthen the body and promote health.

In herbal therapy for health maintenance, medicinal substances are used to supplement deficiencies and regulate the body. Qi-deficient individuals are supplemented with qi, blood-deficient individuals are nourished with blood, yin-deficient individuals are nourished with yin, and yang-deficient individuals are tonified with yang. By replenishing deficiencies and enhancing abundance, the body's vitality is strengthened, leading to robust health and longevity. Typically, symptoms of stagnation and congestion of qi, blood, and phlegm are predominant in those with actual deficiencies.

The purpose of herbal supplementation is to harmonize yin and yang, and it should be done in moderation, avoiding excessive or blind supplementation. Excessive supplementation can lead to imbalances of yin and yang, causing further harm to the body. For example, although someone may have qi deficiency, blindly supplementing with large doses of qi tonics without considering other factors can lead to qi stagnation, resulting in symptoms such as chest and abdominal fullness and disruption of qi movement.

Herbal supplementation should follow a gradual process and should not be rushed. If this principle is not understood, rushing the process may not only be ineffective but also harmful.

Research has shown that many traditional Chinese medicines have effects on promoting, inhibiting, and regulating immune function, thus contributing to disease prevention and longevity. For example, sea cucumber, garlic, sand lily, poria cocos, and cortex phellodendri can activate central immune organs including the spleen and thymus. Solomon's seal, Chinese wolfberry, lily bulb, shiitake mushroom, and cottonseed can increase the percentage of peripheral lymphocytes. Astragalus, ginseng, eleuthero, ligustrum, eclipta, white atractylodes, mulberry, kiwifruit, and dandelion can enhance the conversion rate of peripheral blood lymphocytes.

Cordyceps, panax notoginseng, ginseng, and ophiopogon have effects on improving nucleic acid metabolism. Royal jelly, bee pollen, gelatin, deer antler, and placenta can promote cell regeneration.

Atractylodes, acorus calamus, poria cocos, lingzhi mushroom, cyperus rotundus, and cordyceps have sedative effects. Pearl, musk, antelope horn, and gastrodia elata have anticonvulsant effects, effectively alleviating imbalances in the nervous system. Medicines acting on the cardiovascular system, such as salvia miltiorrhiza, peony, chuanxiong, pumpkin, allium, ginseng, lingzhi, hawthorn, musk, and rehmannia, have significant effects on dilating coronary arteries, reducing peripheral vascular resistance, decreasing myocardial oxygen consumption, increasing cardiac output, and inhibiting platelet aggregation. Medicines acting on the urinary system, such as placenta, eucommia ulmoides, poria cocos, ginseng, and plantain seed, can effectively improve and regulate kidney function.

Medications acting on the respiratory system, such as Radix Glehniae, Cordyceps sinensis, almonds, tea leaves, asarum, bufonis venenum, and honey, have significant effects on preventing and treating chronic bronchitis and emphysema in the elderly. Medications acting on the digestive system, such as white atractylodes, gentiana scabra, musk, schisandra chinensis, rhubarb, hawthorn, and bupleurum, all contribute to the relief and functional recovery of digestive tract and gland diseases in the elderly.

Blood-activating and stasis-resolving medications regulate immune function, enhance disease resistance, improve metabolism, and reduce blood cholesterol levels. These medications not only have certain therapeutic effects on vascular diseases, connective tissue diseases, hemorrhagic diseases, and immune diseases but also play a role in disease prevention and health maintenance in many aspects. Particularly, they have significant effects on improving microcirculation disorders, enhancing myocardial blood supply and oxygenation, preventing thrombosis, dissolving thrombi, preventing atherosclerosis, reducing blood coagulation, decreasing fibrinogen deposition, as well as exerting anti-inflammatory and anti-infection effects. Proper use of blood-activating and stasis-resolving medications according to the physiological characteristics of the elderly can be highly beneficial for delaying aging.

Why do elderly people's hair turn white easily?

THE KIDNEY CHANNEL of the Foot-Shaoyin meridian is responsible for nourishing the bone marrow, and its essence manifests in the hair. When blood and Qi are abundant, the Kidney Qi is strong, leading to a rich bone marrow and lustrous black hair. Conversely, when blood and Qi are deficient, the Kidney Qi weakens, resulting in depleted bone marrow and causing the hair at the temples to turn white.

Under normal circumstances, the hair follicles and roots are richly supplied with blood vessels for nourishment, facilitating the synthesis of melanin granules. When there is a disruption in the synthesis of melanin granules or when they cannot be transported to the hair, white hair occurs.

After the age of 40, the body gradually undergoes aging, and the hair is more prone to turning white. Additionally, cognitive decline, forgetfulness, insomnia, and even emotional and psychological symptoms may occur. The main reason is the weakening of cardiovascular function and the impaired circulation of Qi and blood.

Individuals engaged in mental labor are often in a state of excessive brain use and high mental stress. Combined with unhealthy lifestyles and the influence of emotions and stress, people are more likely to develop premature graying of the hair.

From a medical perspective, the slowing of blood flow, reduction in the number of capillaries, decline in tissue cell function, and changes in membrane permeability lead to a decrease in cellular respiratory activity and a reduced utilization rate of oxygen.

Nutritional deficiencies in the subcutaneous blood vessels can cause hair thinning and hair loss; disturbances in melanin synthesis can result in graying of hair and beard; decreased skin elasticity, reduced subcutaneous fat, and decreased intracellular water content can lead to sagging skin and wrinkles.

The kidneys of elderly individuals undergo atrophy, leading to reduced renal blood flow, decreased glomerular filtration rate, and diminished renal tubular reabsorption capacity, resulting in renal dysfunction.

Hair loss is a common symptom in middle-aged and elderly individuals. In traditional Chinese medicine, the kidneys govern the hair, and hair growth relies on kidney essence and blood. Therefore, treatment should focus on nourishing the liver and kidneys and replenishing Qi and blood.

A formula containing wolfberry fruit, dodder seed, mulberry fruit, fleeceflower root, salvia root, astragalus root, angelica, and arborvitae seed is an ideal method for hair care.

Cooking porridge with wolfberry fruit, fleeceflower root, prepared rehmannia root, mountain hawthorn fruit, black soybeans, and black sesame seeds has a hair-darkening effect and promotes hair growth.

Nutrition for the elders in four seasons

IN ALL FOUR SEASONS of the year, there are changes in climate - spring warmth, summer heat, autumn coolness, and winter coldness. These variations in weather can have different effects on the human body. Therefore, it's important to adjust the nutritional structure of the body according to the seasons, paying attention to scientific dietary habits and supplementation methods for each season, and arranging meals reasonably. In spring, it is advisable to eat lightly; in summer, it is advisable to eat sweet and cool foods; in autumn, due to dryness and heat, it is advisable to eat foods that generate fluids; and in winter, it is advisable to eat warm foods. Adapting dietary habits to the four seasons is particularly important for the elderly.

Spring

SPRING IS THE SEASON of growth and renewal for all things. In early spring, the temperature remains relatively cold, and the body needs to expend energy to maintain its basic temperature. It is important to consume high-quality protein foods such as eggs, fish, shrimp, beef, chicken, rabbit meat, and soy products. Additionally, foods like soybeans, sesame seeds, peanuts, and walnuts should be chosen to replenish energy substances promptly.

During the transition from cold to warm weather, there are significant temperature changes, and bacteria, viruses, and other microorganisms begin to proliferate, becoming more active and easily invading the human body, leading to illness. Therefore, it is important to consume sufficient vitamins and minerals in the diet. Fresh vegetables like bok choy, rapeseed, bell peppers, and tomatoes, as well as citrus fruits like oranges and lemons, should be included. Carrots, amaranth, and other yellow-green vegetables, rich in vitamin A, can protect and strengthen the mucous membranes of the upper respiratory tract and respiratory epithelial cells, thereby resisting various pathogenic factors.

Chronic bronchitis in the elderly is prone to flare-ups in spring. Dietary prevention and treatment methods involve consuming foods that can dispel phlegm, invigorate the spleen, nourish the kidneys, and strengthen the lungs. Examples include loquat, oranges, pears, lotus seeds, lilies, dates, walnuts, and honey, which can help alleviate symptoms.

Summer

THE HOT SUMMER IS THE season when the body consumes the most energy. It is necessary to replenish fluids and nutrients in a timely manner. The diet should be light and refreshing to stimulate the appetite. When planning meals, attention should be paid to the color, aroma, and taste of the food to enhance appetite. For example, one can consume more cold dishes, salted duck eggs, salted eggs, marinated eggs, tofu, sesame paste, mung beans, fresh vegetables, and fruits.

Foods with heat-clearing and heat-relieving effects include amaranth, water shield, malan head (a type of aquatic vegetable), eggplant, fresh lotus root, mung bean sprouts, luffa, cucumber, winter melon, loofah, and watermelon. Tomatoes and watermelons are particularly noteworthy as they not only relieve thirst but also have nourishing effects.

In summer, the high temperature makes people prefer coolness. Therefore, the diet should focus on clearing heat. Clearing heat means consuming primarily cooling foods, such as barley, wheat, mung beans, lilies, sugar, cucumbers, spinach, Chinese cabbage, bean sprouts, celery, watermelon radish, bamboo shoots, eggplant, water chestnuts, rabbit meat, duck meat, lamb liver, milk, eggs, and fresh fruits. Regular consumption of these foods can help clear heat, relieve summer heat, and invigorate the spleen.

Summer is the season of dampness and heat. Elderly people with spleen deficiency should choose nourishing foods that are gentle in nature, help strengthen the spleen and stomach, dispel dampness, and are not greasy. Common options include adzuki beans, coix seeds, which can be cooked until soft and eaten with sugar, and soups like winter melon soup, lily soup, red date soup, and mung bean soup, which help relieve heat, quench thirst, and nourish the body.

In summer, the high temperature increases the risk of food contamination by bacteria, so it is best to avoid eating leftover rice and vegetables. If eaten, they must be thoroughly reheated. Fruits and melons should be washed and peeled before consumption. When making cold dishes, vegetables must be thoroughly washed.

Autumn

AUTUMN IS THE SEASON when fruits ripen, and there is a wide variety of melons, fruits, and leguminous vegetables available. As the temperature gradually cools down and the body's energy consumption decreases, appetite begins to increase. However, the autumn climate is dry, so it is advisable to consume foods that nourish yin, clear heat, moisten dryness, quench thirst, and calm the mind. Foods such as sesame, honey, tremella mushroom, and dairy products, which have moisturizing effects, are suitable choices.

Tremella mushroom and lily combination have the effect of nourishing and moisturizing, invigorating the spleen, and replenishing qi. Tremella mushroom nourishes yin, moistens the lungs, nourishes the stomach, and generates fluids. Lily nourishes lung yin, moistens lung dryness, and calms the mind.

Autumn is a good season for elderly people and those with chronic diseases to engage in nourishing food therapy. Foods suitable for nourishing include bamboo shoots, pumpkin, lotus seeds, longan, black sesame seeds, red dates, and walnuts. Patients with weak spleen and stomach and poor digestion can consume lotus seeds, Chinese yam, and mung beans, which help invigorate the spleen and stomach.

Especially Chinese yam, which has a sweet taste and contains various nutrients such as fat, protein, mucilage, and vitamins, has the effects of nourishing and strengthening the body and aiding digestion.

Walnuts have a sweet taste, are neutral and warm in nature, and have the effects of nourishing the brain, kidneys, and combating fatigue. For elderly people with weak constitution, they can prepare porridge with glutinous rice, raisins, walnut kernels, melon seeds, white fruit kernels, lotus seeds, longan meat, red bean paste, cooked Chinese yam, small red dates, green plums, and osmanthus flowers.

Winter

IN WINTER, THE CLIMATE is cold, and yin energy prevails while yang energy declines. The cold temperature affects the body's physiological functions and appetite. The cold climate of winter affects the body's endocrine system, leading to increased secretion of hormones such as thyroxine and adrenaline, which promote and accelerate the breakdown of protein, fat, and carbohydrates, the three major sources of heat nutrients, to increase the body's ability to withstand the cold. This leads to excessive loss of body heat, requiring timely replenishment.

For elderly individuals, it is important to focus on high-quality protein sources such as lean meat, eggs, fish, dairy products, legumes, and their derivatives. These foods not only facilitate digestion and absorption but also contain essential amino acids, providing high nutritional value and enhancing the body's ability to withstand cold and disease.

Elderly individuals often lack elements such as potassium, calcium, sodium, and iron due to factors affecting digestion, absorption, and metabolism. Therefore, they should consume foods rich in calcium, iron, sodium, potassium, and other nutrients, such as shrimp, shrimp shells, sesame paste, pork liver, and bananas.

Since green leafy vegetables are relatively scarce in winter, it is advisable to consume more starchy foods such as sweet potatoes and potatoes. Additionally, radishes, carrots, and other root vegetables can be eaten more often. Boiled radish with eggs has a good effect in preventing and treating bronchial cough and asthma.

In winter, dietary supplementation should provide foods rich in protein, vitamins, and easy-to-digest nutrients. Options include grains and legumes such as japonica rice, indica rice, corn, wheat, soybeans, and peas; vegetables like leeks, cilantro, garlic, radishes, and cauliflower; meats such as lamb, dog meat, beef, chicken, eels, carp, grass carp, ribbon fish, and shrimp; fruits such as oranges, coconuts, pineapples, lychees, and longans.

For elderly individuals with weak constitution, regularly consuming stewed chicken, lean meat, tendon, and drinking milk, soy milk, etc., can enhance their physique. Lamb and beef are excellent choices for winter nourishment for the elderly, as they have the benefits of tonifying qi, relieving thirst, strengthening tendons and bones, and nourishing the spleen and stomach. White radish has the effects of resolving stagnation, clearing phlegm and heat, detoxifying, relieving flatulence, and harmonizing the middle, and can be cooked together with beef or mutton.

Elderly individuals with hyperlipidemia can regularly consume black sesame mulberry paste. Sweet potatoes have a slimming effect because they contain a large amount of mucin protein, which maintains the elasticity of blood vessel walls, prevents arteriosclerosis, and reduces subcutaneous fat. Therefore, eating fresh sweet potatoes can prevent obesity, lower cholesterol levels, and prevent cardiovascular diseases.

In conclusion, throughout the four seasons, there are many Chinese medicinal herbs suitable for elderly individuals to supplement their health and prolong their lives, categorized into four types based on their functions: supplementing qi, nourishing blood, nourishing yin, and supplementing yang.

Herbs for the elderly to supplement qi

GINSENG

Ginseng has a sweet and slightly bitter taste, with a warming nature. It can greatly replenish vital energy, generate fluids to quench thirst, and is particularly suitable for the elderly and those weakened by long illness, offering the benefits of lightening the body and prolonging life when consumed over time. A decoction made solely from ginseng, known as Duxin Tang, can benefit qi and secure against collapse. It is especially beneficial for the elderly and the frail, strengthening the body and combating aging when consumed over a long period.

Astragalus

Astragalus has a sweet taste and a slightly warm nature. It can replenish qi and lift yang, strengthen the Wei (defensive) energy and consolidate the exterior, promote diuresis to reduce edema, and nourish the five organs. Long-term use can strengthen bones and the body, and treat various types of qi deficiency. In the Qing dynasty court's healthcare practices, astragalus was frequently used to supplement the middle qi and nourish blood. Astragalus can enhance the body's resistance, regulate blood pressure and immune function, and improve coronary circulation and heart function.

Poria

Poria has a sweet and bland taste with a neutral property. It is known for strengthening the spleen and stomach, calming the mind and spirit, and promoting diuresis to resolve dampness. Its medicinal properties are mild, benefiting the heart and spleen, promoting water metabolism without being too harsh, and can both support the body's fundamental energy and eliminate pathogenic factors.

Poria not only enhances the human body's immune function but also improves the body's disease resistance and has a strong anti-cancer effect, truly making it an excellent choice for prolonging life and enhancing health.

Chinese Yam

Chinese yam has a sweet taste and a neutral nature. It has the functions of tonifying the spleen, nourishing the lungs, strengthening the kidneys, and enriching essence. Therefore, for middle-aged and elderly people who are weak and prone to illness, regularly consuming Chinese yam can bring many benefits. It is beneficial for conditions such as senile diabetes and chronic nephritis.

Coix seed

Coix seed has a sweet and bland taste, with a cool nature. It is used for sudden cramps of the tendons, inability to stretch or bend, rheumatic arthralgia, and long-term consumption can lighten the body and replenish qi. Coix seed has the effects of tonifying the spleen, nourishing the lungs, and promoting diuresis.

Coix seed is a medicinal food that can be used as a staple food. It has been recorded in historical documents and has been used up to the present day. Coix seed can be washed and cooked with glutinous rice to make porridge, or it can be cooked alone to make porridge. It has the effects of tonifying the spleen and stomach, promoting diuresis, and resisting cancerous tumors.

Herbs for the elderly to nourish blood

Shu Di Huang

Shu di huang has a sweet taste and a slightly warm nature. It nourishes the bone marrow, promotes muscle growth, generates essence and blood, supplements insufficiency of the five viscera, promotes blood circulation, benefits the ears and eyes, and darkens hair. This herb has the function of nourishing blood and nourishing yin.

For those with blood deficiency and insufficient kidney essence, it can nourish blood, nourish yin, nourish the kidneys, and replenish essence. It has excellent effects in strengthening the heart, diuresis, and lowering blood sugar.

He Shou Wu

He shou wu has a bitter-sweet taste and a slightly astringent nature, with a warm property. It benefits qi and blood, darkens hair, and enhances complexion. Long-term consumption strengthens tendons and bones, nourishes essence and marrow, and prolongs life without aging. This herb has the functions of nourishing essence and blood, astringing essence to stop emissions, and nourishing the liver and kidneys.

The longevity and anti-aging effects of he shou wu are achieved by strengthening the nerves, enhancing cardiac function, lowering blood lipids, and relieving arteriosclerosis, thereby enhancing the body's constitution.

Longan Flesh

Longan flesh has a sweet taste and a warm nature. It has the function of nourishing the heart, spleen, and qi and blood. Longan flesh porridge nourishes the heart, calms the mind, strengthens the spleen, and nourishes the blood. It has a certain therapeutic effect on neurogenic palpitations.

Donkey-hide Gelatin

Donkey-hide gelatin has a sweet taste and a neutral nature. It has the functions of nourishing blood and nourishing yin, stopping bleeding and securing the fetus, promoting urination, and moistening the large intestine.

It has the effect of accelerating the production of red blood cells and hemoglobin, promoting blood coagulation, and is therefore good at replenishing blood and stopping bleeding.

Zi He Che

Zi He Che has a sweet and salty taste and a slightly warm nature. It has the effects of nourishing blood, replenishing qi, and nourishing essence.

Zi He Che can promote the development of mammary glands and uterus; it can enhance the body's resistance and has immunomodulatory and anti-allergic effects.

Herbs for the elderly to nourish yin

WOLFBERRY (GOJI BERRY)

Wolfberry has a sweet taste and a neutral nature. It nourishes the blood and supplements deficiencies, and is effective in reducing fever. It specializes in nourishing the kidneys, moistening the lungs, generating fluids, and replenishing qi. It is an essential medicine for replenishing the true yin of the liver and kidneys, as well as for replenishing internal heat due to fatigue. It has the effects of nourishing the kidneys, moistening the lungs, and clearing the liver to improve vision.

Wolfberry inhibits the deposition of fat in liver cells, preventing fatty liver, and promoting the regeneration of liver cells.

Polygonatum Odoratum (Yu Zhu)

Polygonatum odoratum has a sweet taste and a neutral nature. It can nourish yin and moisten the lungs, relieve irritability, and quench thirst, making it particularly suitable for elderly individuals with yin deficiency.

It has the effect of lowering blood sugar and strengthening the heart. It has a certain effect on diabetic patients and patients with palpitations. It is not greasy in nature and can be applied to conditions of insufficient body fluids. However, it should be used with caution or avoided in cases of gastric distention, dampness, or phlegm excess.

Solomon's Seal

Solomon's Seal (Polygonatum) tastes sweet and is neutral in nature. It benefits the spleen and stomach, moistens the heart and lungs, and replenishes essence and marrow. It is beneficial for cases of both qi and yin deficiency, fatigue, dry mouth, and lack of saliva.

Solomon's Seal has a blood pressure-lowering effect and can also help prevent arteriosclerosis and fatty liver infiltration to a certain extent.

Mulberry Fruit

Mulberry fruit tastes bitter and is cold in nature. It can nourish the liver and kidneys, enrich yin and blood, and, with long-term use, can darken hair and brighten the eyes.

It is used clinically for anemia, nervous debility, diabetes, and yin-deficient hypertension.

Ligustrum

Ligustrum (Privet) fruit tastes slightly sweet and bitter and is neutral. It can nourish the liver and kidneys, strengthen yin, and brighten the eyes. It is nourishing without being greasy, but its nature is slightly cool, so it should be used with caution in cases of spleen and stomach deficiency, diarrhea, and yang deficiency.

Ligustrum contains fatty oils, including palmitic acid, oleic acid, and linolenic acid. It has cardiotonic and diuretic effects and can also be used for lymphatic tuberculosis, pulmonary tuberculosis, and fever.

Herbs for the elderly to supplement yang

DODDER SEED

Dodder seed tastes sweet and slightly spicy, and is slightly warm in nature. It has the effects of nourishing the liver and kidneys, nourishing essence and marrow, strengthening tendons and bones, and enhancing qi and strength.

Deer Antler

Deer antler tastes sweet and salty, and is warm in nature. It has the effects of tonifying kidney yang, nourishing essence and blood, and strengthening tendons and bones.

Deer antler can reduce fatigue, improve work efficiency, and enhance appetite and sleep. It can promote the regeneration of red blood cells, hemoglobin, and reticulocytes, and accelerate the healing of wounds, fractures, and ulcers. It is a good general tonic.

Cistanche

Cistanche tastes sweet and salty, and is warm in nature. It has the effects of tonifying the kidney and assisting yang, moistening the intestines and promoting bowel movements. It also has the functions of lowering blood pressure, strengthening the heart, enhancing physical strength, and increasing the body's resistance.

Eucommia Bark

Eucommia bark tastes sweet and is warm in nature. It has the effects of tonifying the liver and kidneys, strengthening tendons and bones, and stabilizing pregnancy. It also has sedative and blood pressure-lowering effects.

Chapter 4
Dietary Management of Common Diseases in the Elderly

Dietary Management of Hypertension

Hypertension is a clinical syndrome characterized by elevated arterial blood pressure and is one of the common diseases in the elderly. It is closely related to factors such as genetics, long-term psychological stress, obesity, excessive salt intake, and smoking.

Animal fats contain high levels of saturated fatty acids, which can raise cholesterol levels, increase the risk of thrombosis, and raise the incidence of hypertension-related strokes. On the other hand, vegetable oils contain higher levels of unsaturated fatty acids, which can prolong platelet aggregation time, inhibit thrombosis formation, lower blood pressure, and prevent strokes. Therefore, it is advisable to consume more vegetable oils and choose foods low in saturated fatty acids and cholesterol, such as vegetables, fruits, whole grains, fish, poultry, lean meat, and low-fat dairy products.

Hypertensive patients should control their energy intake by limiting the consumption of staple foods and fats, and avoiding or minimizing high-energy foods such as sweets, snacks, sweetened beverages, and fried foods. Reduce the amount of salt used in cooking and minimize consumption of salt-preserved foods such as pickles. Increase intake of seafood appropriately, such as seaweed, laver, and marine fish.

Dietary Management of Hyperlipidemia

HYPERLIPIDEMIA REFERS to elevated levels of cholesterol or triglycerides in the blood, or both. It can be caused by other diseases such as diabetes, chronic kidney disease, gout, alcoholism, etc. It is closely related to the formation of atherosclerosis and is one of the main risk factors for triggering coronary heart disease.

Patients should limit their dietary intake of cholesterol. Foods high in cholesterol should be avoided, such as animal brains, liver, kidneys, crab roe, fish roe, egg yolks, century eggs, etc. Overweight or obese individuals should pay particular attention to moderation. Foods high in pure sugars and sweets should be avoided.

Many foods have lipid-lowering effects, such as garlic, eggplant, shiitake mushrooms, wood ear mushrooms, onions, seaweed, soybeans, tea, fish, sesame oil, corn oil, peanut oil, and other vegetable oils. Other foods like hawthorn, celery, winter melon, coarse oats, apples, etc., also have varying degrees of lipid-lowering effects.

Dietary Management of Coronary Heart Disease

CORONARY HEART DISEASE is a cardiac condition caused by atherosclerosis of the coronary arteries, leading to insufficient blood supply to the heart muscle. The primary clinical manifestations of coronary heart disease are angina and arrhythmias due to myocardial ischemia and hypoxia. In severe cases, it can lead to myocardial infarction, causing extensive necrosis of the heart muscle and endangering life.

The factors contributing to the onset of coronary heart disease mainly include hypertension, hypercholesterolemia, and smoking; followed by obesity, diabetes, and psychological factors, which are directly related to the patient's emotions.

Patients should control their intake of staple foods and fats, ensuring a supply of fresh vegetables and fruits to provide vitamins and an appropriate amount of dietary fiber. Try to minimize the use of foods high in cholesterol, such as animal liver, brain, kidneys, fish roe, as well as high fatty acid foods like fatty meats, animal fats, butter, and cream. It is beneficial for the prevention and treatment of coronary heart disease to choose more legumes and soy products.

Increase the intake of marine products, such as kelp, seaweed, and jellyfish, to provide the body with abundant iodine. Opt for more aquatic fish. Foods like winter melon, radish, honey, and hawthorn can also be chosen.

Dietary Management of Stroke

STROKE, OR CEREBROVASCULAR accident, is a common and frequently occurring disease among middle-aged and elderly individuals. The clinical manifestations often include sudden onset of consciousness disorders and limb paralysis, mainly in elderly individuals with hypertension or atherosclerosis.

From a preventive perspective, the dietary principles for preventing cerebrovascular accidents are consistent with those for hypertension, atherosclerosis, and hyperlipidemia patients.

Food choices for patients may include milk, soy milk, thick rice soup, diluted lotus root powder, diluted fried noodles, milk substitutes, powdered milk, malted milk, egg powder, fish powder, meat powder, meat broth, chicken broth, sucrose, maltose, refined vegetable oil, vegetable juice, fruit juice, etc. To ensure dietary balance, efforts should be made to diversify food choices.

Dietary Management of Chronic Bronchitis, Emphysema, and Cor Pulmonale

CHRONIC BRONCHITIS has complex causes. Middle-aged and elderly individuals with the condition often experience gradually worsening difficulty in breathing, shortness of breath, and dyspnea after exertion. Symptoms worsen during cold seasons due to respiratory infections. Long-term repeated coughing causes alveolar expansion, increased pressure, and increased cardiac burden, eventually leading to cor pulmonale.

Patients should have sufficient daily intake of protein from various sources such as fish, poultry, lean meat, eggs, dairy, and legumes.

It is important to choose foods rich in vitamins A, B, and C, such as liver, egg yolks, green leafy and yellow vegetables, fresh oranges, oranges, and tangerines. This helps maintain normal function of tracheal mucosal epithelial cells and enhances the body's resistance. Foods like wood ear mushrooms, peanuts, loofah, bamboo shoots, radishes, lotus roots, walnuts, pears, honey, and seaweed have phlegm-clearing and lung-moistening functions.

Avoid overly stimulating and extreme hot or cold foods, such as alcohol, tea, onions, chili peppers, etc., and quit smoking.

Dietary Management of Chronic Gastritis

CHRONIC GASTRITIS IS a chronic inflammatory lesion of the gastric mucosa caused by various factors, and its incidence increases with age. Most patients may experience varying degrees of indigestion symptoms, loss of appetite or aversion to food, and a feeling of fullness or pain in the upper abdomen, which often occurs immediately after eating. Some patients may also experience symptoms such as emaciation, anemia, and glossitis. Those with excessive gastric acid secretion may experience heartburn and acid reflux.

Staple foods such as soft rice, bread, steamed buns, buns, and dumplings are suitable choices. Milk, cream, starch, vegetables, and well-cooked lean meat, which do not stimulate gastric acid secretion, are suitable for patients with high acidity gastritis.

Fresh vegetables and fruits with low fiber content, such as winter melon, cucumber, tomatoes, potatoes, spinach, Chinese cabbage, apples, pears, bananas, and oranges, are relatively suitable for gastritis patients to consume.

Dietary Management of Hepatitis

HEPATITIS VIRUSES CAN be classified into various types clinically. The main clinical manifestations of viral hepatitis include loss of appetite, aversion to oily foods, nausea, vomiting, bloating, diarrhea or constipation. During the acute phase, patients may also experience fever, headache, dizziness, general weakness, and insomnia. Physical examination may reveal hepatomegaly and tenderness in the liver area. Patients often complain of discomfort or pain in the liver area, and some may present with jaundice. Liver function tests may show elevated transaminases.

Nutrition and diet play a significant role in the treatment of hepatitis. Generally, high-quality protein foods such as fish, lean meat, eggs, dairy products, and soy products should be prioritized, and staple foods should be ensured.

The intake of fresh vegetables and fruits should be increased. It is advisable to consume fewer or no fried foods and other high-fat foods. Spicy and other irritating foods should be consumed cautiously. Alcohol consumption should be strictly prohibited.

Dietary Management of Gout

GOUT IS PRIMARILY CAUSED by allergic inflammation in the joints and surrounding soft tissues, with a tendency to recur. Acute attacks of arthritis often occur at night, with sudden and intense pain in the big toe, limb joints, fingers, and other areas. The affected joints show signs of redness, swelling, heat, and pain. In the chronic phase, attacks are frequent, lasting longer, and involving more joints. Gouty tophi erosion of bone can lead to skeletal deformities. Patients may also have chronic renal insufficiency, coronary heart disease, and cerebral arteriosclerosis.

It is advisable to choose foods that are either low in purines or purine-free, such as refined flour, rice, soda crackers, steamed buns, bread, dairy and dairy products, eggs, various oils and fats, fruits, dried fruits, sugar, and candies. With the exception of a few vegetables like cauliflower and spinach, most vegetables such as carrots, celery, cabbage, cucumbers, eggplants, tomatoes, zucchinis, and potatoes are suitable.

High-purine foods include pancreas, anchovies, liver, kidneys, brains, meat broth, chicken broth, poultry and livestock meats, carp, eels, bass, mullet, sardines, ham, shellfish, and lentils. Consumption of these foods should be strictly limited.

Dietary Management of Diabetes

DURING THE SYMPTOMATIC phase, clinical manifestations of diabetes include polydipsia, polyphagia, polyuria, weight loss, fatigue, emaciation, itching skin, limb soreness, decreased sexual function, and constipation. Diabetes patients are prone to complications such as acute infections, pulmonary tuberculosis, arteriosclerosis, retinal and renal microvascular lesions, and neurological disorders. It is generally believed that these symptoms result from insufficient insulin, leading to metabolic disorders of carbohydrates, fats, and proteins in the body.

Diabetic patients should strictly limit their food intake. High-quality protein foods with low cholesterol content can be chosen, such as dairy products, eggs, soy products, fish, and lean meats, while the consumption of animal liver and other viscera should be restricted.

Increasing dietary fiber intake is recommended. In addition to coarse grains, vegetables, and fruits high in fiber, foods such as bean curd, pectin, bran, algin, and konjac can also be consumed.

It is advisable to avoid foods such as white sugar, chocolate, honey, preserves, syrup, fructose, sugary beverages, and sweet pastries.

Anti-Cancer Foods

CANCER BELONGS TO A category of diseases characterized by deficiency in righteousness and excess in evil, where evil overwhelms righteousness. Therefore, the basic principle of treatment is to support righteousness and expel evil, employing both tonification and elimination strategies. Tonification focuses on rectifying deficiencies based on different emphasis on deficiency, combined with the main lesions of the organs, and adopting methods such as tonifying Qi, blood, Yin, and Yang. Expelling evil mainly targets lesions, utilizing methods like promoting Qi circulation, resolving phlegm and nodules, promoting blood circulation and removing blood stasis, clearing heat and detoxification.

Prevention is crucial for reducing the incidence of cancer. Strengthening dietary regulation, regulating emotions, and paying attention to rest are beneficial for the recovery from cancer.

The basic characteristic of cancer is the occurrence of abnormal masses in visceral tissues. The formation of these masses is often attributed to the intertwining of Qi stagnation, phlegm stagnation, dampness obstruction, blood stasis, and toxin accumulation over time, resulting in tangible masses. Cancer patients often have a weakened constitution, and the progression of cancer consumes the body's Qi, blood, essence, and fluids. Therefore, in the middle and late stages, patients often experience deficiencies in Qi and blood, as well as the transformation of Yin and Yang deficiencies.

Qi deficiency is mainly due to dietary imbalance, inadequate essence from food and drink, and insufficient sources of Qi; or due to chronic illness, aging and weakness, and excessive fatigue, leading to weakened organ function and insufficient Qi generation.

Blood deficiency is often caused by excessive blood loss, weak spleen and stomach, poor nutrition, chronic unresolved illness, and disorders in blood generation. Due to the deficiency of nutritive blood, the organs and meridians are inadequately nourished, manifesting symptoms such as dizziness, fatigue, pale complexion, and lackluster lips and nails.

Dietary imbalance is one of the significant factors leading to cancer transformation. Damp stagnation, due to external factors or internal injuries, poor diet, and other reasons, leads to dysfunction of the lungs, spleen, and kidneys, disrupting water metabolism and causing fluid retention and dampness issues. Depending on the site of the lesion, there are various clinical manifestations. When dampness is trapped in the middle jiao affecting the spleen and stomach, it can lead to loss of appetite, dullness, abdominal bloating, and diarrhea.

Below are some foods that are beneficial for the prevention and treatment of cancer.

Asparagus

ASPARAGUS HAS CERTAIN therapeutic effects on hypertension, heart disease, tachycardia, fatigue, edema, cystitis, difficulty urinating, and other conditions. In recent years, American scholars have discovered that asparagus has the function of preventing the spread of cancer cells, and it has special therapeutic effects on lymphoma, bladder cancer, lung cancer, skin cancer, kidney stones, and other conditions. Asparagus can also treat leukemia, which has been recognized worldwide.

Garlic

GARLIC IN RECENT YEARS, the anti-cancer effects of garlic have been widely recognized. Effective components such as lipid-soluble volatile oils in garlic have the function of activating macrophages and enhancing immunity, thereby improving the body's resistance. Garlic can also inhibit the growth of nitrate-reducing bacteria in the stomach, thereby reducing the production of nitrites in the stomach due to bacterial action.

In addition, garlic contains trace elements such as selenium and germanium, as well as various anti-cancer substances, so eating garlic regularly can prevent the occurrence of gastric cancer and esophageal cancer. Garlic also has some unique functions. During the summer and autumn seasons when intestinal infectious diseases are prevalent, or during the winter and spring seasons when respiratory infectious diseases are prevalent, consuming 1-2 cloves of raw garlic daily can prevent diseases. For conditions such as colds, bronchitis, pharyngitis, tonsillitis, etc., holding 2-3 cloves of raw garlic in the mouth and changing them 3-4 times a day can also be effective. Enema with garlic infusion can expel hookworms, roundworms, and pinworms, and can also treat dysentery and diarrhea.

Crushing fresh garlic into a paste and filling it into cavities can relieve pain from tooth decay. Applying garlic juice to the affected area can treat athlete's foot. Placing a clean gauze strip soaked in garlic juice into the vagina can treat vaginal trichomoniasis.

Cabbage

ACCORDING TO ANCIENT medical books, cabbage has the effects of promoting digestion, relieving chest discomfort, sobering up, aiding digestion, and regulating bowel movements.

In recent years, medical scientists have found that fiber can prevent colon cancer. Cabbage contains a relatively high amount of fiber, which is beneficial for cancer prevention. Additionally, Chinese cabbage contains a considerable amount of the trace element zinc. Zinc promotes blood production, plays an important role in wound healing, and is associated with anti-aging effects. Regular consumption of cabbage is also beneficial for preventing atherosclerosis and cardiovascular diseases.

Shiitake Mushrooms

SHIITAKE MUSHROOMS contain abundant dietary fiber, and regular consumption can lower cholesterol levels in the blood, prevent atherosclerosis, and be effective in preventing cerebral hemorrhage, heart disease, obesity, and diabetes. In recent years, American scientists have found that shiitake mushrooms significantly enhance the body's anti-cancer capabilities. Shiitake mushrooms also have antiviral properties against the common cold virus. Shiitake mushrooms have a cold nature and a slightly bitter taste, which is beneficial for nourishing the liver and strengthening the stomach. Ancient scholars have long discovered that mushrooms can improve brain cell function.

Carrots

CAROTENE, FOUND IN carrots, is crucial for maintaining the normal function of epithelial cells, preventing respiratory infections, promoting growth and development, and participating in the synthesis of rhodopsin. Carrots have a significant role in cancer prevention and treatment. Studies have shown that individuals lacking vitamin A have more than twice the cancer incidence rate compared to healthy individuals. Consuming a certain amount of carrots daily can greatly benefit cancer prevention.

Lignin in carrots also enhances the body's immune capacity against cancer and indirectly kills cancer cells. For people who smoke regularly, drinking half a cup of carrot juice daily can protect the lungs.

Corn

IN RECENT YEARS, SCIENTISTS have discovered new values in corn, finding it has a good preventive and therapeutic effect on modern civilization diseases such as hypertension, arteriosclerosis, coronary heart disease, and cancer.

Corn is rich in glutathione, a cancer-fighting agent. This agent can bind with various external chemical carcinogens in the body, neutralizing their toxicity, and then expelling them through the digestive tract. Coarsely ground corn also contains a large amount of lysine, an amino acid that can not only mitigate the toxic side effects of anticancer drugs but also control tumor growth.

Kiwi

KIWI HAS A SWEET AND sour taste, and it is cold in nature. It is known for its nourishing and strengthening properties, heat-clearing and diuretic effects, as well as its ability to generate fluids and moisturize dryness, and enhance brain function while stopping diarrhea. All parts of the kiwi plant, including its fruit, flowers, leaves, and roots, can be used in medicine. It can be used to treat conditions such as liver and kidney yin deficiency, dryness and heat generating fluids, spleen and stomach qi deficiency, indigestion, and chronic diarrhea. It can also be used to treat conditions like scurvy, allergic purpura, colds, heat toxins, and throat swelling and pain.

Research has shown that fresh kiwi fruit and kiwi juice products not only supplement the body's nutrition but also prevent the formation of carcinogenic substances such as nitrosamines in the body. They can also reduce serum cholesterol and triglyceride levels, significantly preventing and assisting in the treatment of digestive tract cancers, hypertension, and cardiovascular diseases.

Kelp

IN RECENT YEARS, SCIENTISTS have discovered that regularly consuming kelp has a positive effect on the prevention and treatment of cancer. This is because kelp is most famously known for being rich in iodine. When the dietary and drinking water iodine content is low, it can cause simple goiter, which can easily transform into thyroid tumors. A low-iodine diet also promotes hormone-related breast cancer. Therefore, consuming kelp regularly can effectively prevent and treat the occurrence of simple goiter, thereby preventing the aforementioned cancers.

Kelp contains 60% alginates, which are excellent dietary fibers. When consumed by diabetic patients, alginates can delay gastric emptying and passage through the small intestine. This means that even when insulin secretion is reduced, blood sugar levels do not rise, thereby achieving the purpose of treating diabetes. For obese patients, consuming kelp can reduce hunger while absorbing a variety of amino acids and inorganic salts, making it an ideal satiety aid. Additionally, seaweed can promote intestinal peristalsis, ensuring smooth bowel movements and reducing the retention time of feces and toxins in the intestines, thereby preventing the occurrence of rectal cancer.

Round Cabbage

ROUND CABBAGE CONTAINS abundant trace element molybdenum, which has the ability to inhibit the synthesis of carcinogenic nitrosamines, thus possessing certain anti-cancer properties. Currently, as an anti-cancer substance, it, along with cauliflower, kale, and Brussels sprouts, has been included in the anti-cancer diet by scientists worldwide.

Modern medicine and clinical practice have proven that round cabbage also has a wide range of preventive and therapeutic effects. For example, using fresh round cabbage juice to treat gastric and duodenal ulcers can enhance the resistance of the gastrointestinal mucosa epithelium, normalize metabolic processes, and thereby accelerate ulcer healing. The pectin and cellulose contained in round cabbage can bind and inhibit the absorption of cholesterol and bile acids in the intestines, making it beneficial for patients with atherosclerosis, local myocardial ischemia, cholelithiasis, and obesity. Regular consumption of round cabbage also has a good effect on preventing and treating chronic diseases such as hepatitis and cholecystitis.

Lily

LILY HAS A SWEET TASTE and neutral property. It is known for its effectiveness in warming the lungs and relieving coughs, nourishing Yin and clearing heat, calming the mind, and promoting urination. It is particularly beneficial for treating heart and lung diseases. It is suitable for conditions such as lingering heat after febrile diseases, restlessness, palpitations, mental confusion, chronic cough due to pulmonary tuberculosis, hemoptysis, and more.

When used in soups or congee with added tremella fungus, Lily has the ability to nourish Yin and moisten the lungs. If combined with lotus seeds, it can nourish Yin and clear the heart.

In terms of cancer prevention and treatment, Lily is often used to treat lung cancer, nasopharyngeal carcinoma, skin cancer, and other types. For symptoms such as weakness, dry mouth, restlessness, and dry cough with phlegm that occur after radiotherapy for these cancers, cooking Lily with glutinous rice into a congee and adding an appropriate amount of rock sugar or honey before consumption can enhance the body's constitution, inhibit the growth of cancer cells, and alleviate the side effects of radiotherapy. Additionally, applying a mashed mixture of fresh Lily and white sugar to affected areas can have a certain therapeutic effect on bleeding and oozing skin cancer lesions.

Tomato

TOMATO IS THE PREFERRED fruit and vegetable for cancer prevention and treatment. The organic acids such as malic acid and citric acid in tomatoes not only protect the vitamin C content from being destroyed by cooking but also increase gastric acidity, aid digestion, and regulate gastrointestinal function. For those with weak digestion and insufficient gastric acid, consuming tomatoes or drinking tomato juice in moderation can assist in recovery from illness. The fruit acids in tomatoes can also reduce blood cholesterol levels, benefiting those with hyperlipidemia.

According to pharmacological research, tomato juice has a slow effect on lowering blood pressure and diuretic properties, which can be beneficial as an adjunctive treatment for hypertension and kidney disease patients.

In traditional Chinese medicine, tomatoes are considered to have a sour and sweet taste and possess the effects of quenching thirst, invigorating the stomach, promoting digestion, and clearing heat and detoxification. They are effective in treating symptoms such as thirst due to heat-related illnesses, indigestion caused by overeating oily and heavy foods, heatstroke, bitter taste in the mouth due to stomach heat, and symptoms of internal heat. During hot summers when appetite decreases, consuming sugar-coated tomatoes or tomato soup can relieve heat, stimulate appetite, and aid digestion.

Chapter 5
Common Foods and Their Functions in TCM Terms

Pungent and Warm Herbs for Releasing the Exterior

Perilla Leaf

PERILLA LEAF'S MAIN effect is to release the exterior and dispel cold, regulate qi, and harmonize the middle. It can alleviate symptoms of wind-cold common cold, coughing and shortness of breath, morning sickness during pregnancy, promote qi circulation to stabilize pregnancy, and restlessness of the fetus. It can be used to treat abdominal pain and diarrhea caused by poisoning from eating fish and crabs.

Ginger

GINGER CONTAINS VOLATILE oils that can stimulate the secretion of gastric juice and promote digestion, having a stomach-strengthening effect. Ginger excites the vascular movement center and respiratory center. Ginger is a commonly used food for its therapeutic benefits. Young ginger is often used as a daily condiment and for making pickles, while processed older ginger is used in medicine. It is considered a holy medicine for nausea. For stomach cold and pain, ginger can be decocted and mixed with brown sugar, which has a warming stomach and cold-dispelling effect.

Onion

ONIONS CONTAIN PROTEIN, fat, carbohydrates, vitamins A, B, and C, as well as minerals such as calcium, magnesium, and iron. Additionally, they contain volatile oils, with the component allyl sulfide exhibiting strong antibacterial properties.

Furthermore, a compound called onionin extracted from onions is used in the treatment of atherosclerosis and has shown promising results.

Combining the white part of onions with fermented black beans and decocting them together can treat wind-cold common cold.

Onions can also be used to treat bacterial dysentery and kidney stones. People who regularly consume onions, despite having a high-fat diet, tend to have low cholesterol levels and robust health.

Garlic

GARLIC HAS A CERTAIN therapeutic effect on hypertension, atherosclerosis, coronary heart disease, and vascular embolism. It is a health food for the elderly with the above-mentioned conditions.

Eating more onions in the summer and autumn seasons can prevent and treat intestinal infectious diseases caused by Shigella and Escherichia coli. Additionally, onions are rich in spicy volatile oils, which can stimulate the digestive systems of middle-aged and elderly people with low function, promote the secretion of digestive juices, and aid in digestion.

Due to its high volatility, onions can produce gas when consumed, so it is advisable not to consume them excessively to prevent bloating and flatulence.

Cilantro

CILANTRO IS A COMMONLY used seasoning in daily life, with a fragrant aroma that stimulates the appetite. For children with incomplete measles eruption, bathing the body with cilantro decoction can promote peripheral blood circulation and facilitate the eruption of rashes. Consuming cilantro regularly can warm the spleen and stomach, aid digestion, and is suitable for individuals with a cold constitution, weak stomach, or intestinal obstruction.

Pungent and Cold Herbs for Releasing the Exterior

Mulberry Leaf

MULBERRY LEAVES ARE a cooling and blood-nourishing health food. Drinking mulberry leaf tea regularly can clear heat from the lungs and stomach, and cool the liver while nourishing the blood. It is suitable for individuals with a hot constitution or gastrointestinal stagnation. This product is beneficial for the liver and eyes, and can treat symptoms such as feverish cold, red and swollen eyes, and blurry vision.

Chrysanthemum

CHRYSANTHEMUM IS USED to dispel wind and clear heat, soothe the liver and extinguish wind, clear the liver and brighten the eyes, and clear heat and detoxify. It is suitable for early-stage wind-heat colds and febrile diseases, with symptoms such as fever and headache. It can be combined with mulberry leaves or cooked with glutinous rice porridge until nearly done, then boiled briefly with chrysanthemum and sweetened with white sugar for consumption.

Chrysanthemum is a health food for clearing heat and detoxifying, suitable for individuals with a hot constitution, gastrointestinal heat accumulation, and the elderly, especially suitable for consumption during hot summer days. It can be used to make chrysanthemum-filled pastries.

Peppermint

PEPPERMINT IS A HEALTH food for clearing and refreshing the head. It is suitable for individuals with a hot constitution and liver depression and qi stagnation.

When experiencing wind-heat colds or early-stage febrile diseases, finely ground peppermint can be mixed with honey or white sugar to make pills for clearing wind-heat. For sore throat due to wind-heat, it can be combined with balloon flower, or boiled with an appropriate amount of licorice and drank as a tea substitute, serving as a remedy for oral and throat discomfort.

Fermented Black Soybeans

THIS PRODUCT IS MADE from processed soybeans and is commonly used as a seasoning. It is used for wind-cold or wind-heat colds, distention and stuffiness in the epigastrium, poor appetite, sudden diarrhea in typhoid fever, and painful abdominal bloating. Consuming it regularly can regulate spleen and stomach qi, promote fetal health during pregnancy. It is suitable for individuals with spleen and stomach qi stagnation and pregnant women. Common health-preserving recipes include stewed chicken with fermented black soybeans.

Cooling and Heat-clearing Foods

Water Bamboo Shoots

WATER BAMBOO SHOOTS are best when they are thick and tender. They have a cold nature and are suitable for conditions of yin deficiency with internal heat, constipation with dark urine, dry throat, and other heat-related symptoms. They have the ability to clear heat and relieve irritability, and are helpful for constipation, restlessness in the chest, and high blood pressure. For women who have insufficient milk production after childbirth, fresh water bamboo shoots cooked with pig trotters can help promote lactation.

Chinese Toon Leaves

CHINESE TOON LEAVES are a seasonal delicacy. They can be used to make scrambled eggs, pickled with salt, or served cold, all of which have unique flavors. Chinese toon leaves can invigorate the stomach, stop bleeding, reduce inflammation, and kill parasites. They are used to treat conditions such as uterine inflammation, enteritis, dysentery, and urethritis.

Banana

THE AQUEOUS SOLUTION of methanol extract from ripe banana flesh has the effect of inhibiting fungi and bacteria. Bananas are suitable for treating diabetes, fatty diarrhea, and toxic indigestion. They are moist and soft in texture, making them suitable for the elderly, habitual constipation, hypertension, and coronary heart disease patients to eat regularly. However, excessive consumption can lead to gastrointestinal disorders.

Corn

SIMILAR AS MILLET, its main function is to invigorate the spleen and stomach. Corn contains relatively high levels of protein and fat, with protein containing large amounts of glutamic acid, proline, alanine, and arginine, which have nourishing effects. It has a sweet and mild nature, which can invigorate the spleen, benefit the qi, strengthen the spleen, aid digestion, and stop diarrhea. Many postpartum women prefer to eat corn porridge, making it a good food for infants and young children. Corn should not be eaten with almonds, as it can cause nausea and diarrhea if consumed together.

Tea Leaves

TEAS LIKE CAMELLIA sinensis has a bitter and sweet taste, and is cooling in nature. It can generate fluids to quench thirst, clear heat and detoxify, dispel dampness and promote diuresis, aid digestion and stop diarrhea, and clear the mind and refresh the spirit. Tea plants are usually harvested after three years of growth. The best time to pick the tender leaves is around the Qingming Festival, and the quality deteriorates the later the picking time. Due to different processing methods, tea can be categorized into green tea, black tea, etc. Green tea can clear the mind, purge heat, and refresh the lungs and stomach. Black tea can warm the spleen and stomach, and regulate the middle burner. Tea leaves have certain effects in treating radiation damage, protecting hematopoietic function, and increasing white blood cell count. They can also treat dysentery, acute and chronic gastroenteritis, acute infectious hepatitis, and other diseases.

Foods to Clear Heat and Cool Blood

Water Celery

WATER CELERY IS CONSUMED for its tender stems, often used in various dishes during winter and spring, providing a delightful taste. It can clear heat, making it suitable for those with Yin deficiency and excessive heat. There are two types of celery: green-stemmed and white-stemmed, with the former being superior in medicinal efficacy. Celery contains a high amount of iron, making it an excellent choice for patients with iron deficiency anemia.

Eggplant

EGGPLANT IS A VEGETABLE commonly consumed during the summer and autumn seasons. It has the properties of clearing heat, reducing swelling, promoting diuresis, and strengthening the spleen and stomach. It is helpful for conditions such as intestinal wind bleeding, edema, jaundice hepatitis, and loss of appetite. Eggplant has a cold nature, so it is often paired with warm ingredients such as scallions, ginger, garlic, and cilantro when consumed. Individuals with a cold constitution or those suffering from chronic diarrhea should avoid excessive consumption.

Lotus Root

FRESH LOTUS ROOT IS crispy and refreshing, making it an excellent choice for relieving summer heat and quenching thirst. When cooked, it can clear heat, moisten the lungs, cool the blood, promote digestion, stop diarrhea, and solidify semen. It is suitable for various bleeding disorders, including gynecological bleeding, especially during and after febrile diseases.

Lotus nodes stop bleeding, lotus seeds clear heat and calm the mind, lotus stamen solidifies semen and stops bleeding, lotus pods stop bleeding and dissipate stasis, lotus stems promote lactation and widen the chest, lotus leaves clear heat and reduce fever, and lotus stigmas stabilize pregnancy and stop bleeding. Lotus root can also be processed into lotus root powder, which is consumed by mixing it with hot water, and it is commonly used as an ingredient in dishes.

Wood Ear Mushroom

WOOD EAR MUSHROOM IS a fungus that parasitizes on mulberry, locust, willow, elm, and other trees. Its quality varies depending on the type of tree it grows on. Wood ear mushroom is rich in nutrients and is a nourishing and strengthening food, containing a large amount of carbohydrates. Its gelatinous substance can clear the stomach and intestines.

Wood ear mushroom is high in calcium and iron. Its fat content also contains lecithin and cephalin, which can be used in dishes for nourishment and strengthening. Black wood ear mushroom can treat conditions such as continuous bloody dysentery, abdominal pain, mental restlessness, internal and external hemorrhoids, and anemia.

Watermelon

WATERMELON CLEARS HEAT, relieves summer heat, relieves annoyance, quenches thirst, and promotes urination. Watermelon contains malic acid, fructose, glucose, sucrose, various amino acids, carotene, as well as trace elements such as calcium, phosphorus, and potassium, with a high potassium content. Its contained inorganic salts have a diuretic effect, and the contained protease can convert insoluble proteins into soluble ones, which can be used in conjunction with the treatment of acute and chronic nephritis.

Watermelon rind, with its sweet and cool properties, has excellent diuretic and diuretic effects and can be used as an adjunctive treatment for hypertension. However, it is best to consume less if one's spleen and stomach are deficient and cold, or if one experiences loose stools.

Tomato

TOMATOES CAN LOWER blood pressure and increase capillary permeability, have certain anti-inflammatory and diuretic effects, and are beneficial for kidney disease patients. Tomatoes are high in water content and have the functions of clearing heat, detoxifying, generating fluid, and promoting urination. They are helpful for hypertension and retinal hemorrhage.

Tomatoes have an attractive appearance, bright color, abundant juice, thick flesh, and a delicious sweet and sour taste. They are both a vegetable and a fruit, with high nutritional and medicinal value. Due to their slightly cold and sweet taste, they enter the liver, spleen, and stomach meridians, making them have the function of clearing and tonifying.

Tomatoes have a significant preventive effect on prostate cancer, lung cancer, and stomach cancer.

Sugarcane

SUGARCANE IS SWEET, cool, and abundant in juice. It harmonizes the stomach, moistens the intestines, relieves thirst, and alleviates irritability caused by internal heat and thirst. It is suitable for those who often feel hot and thirsty.

The residue of sugarcane, when dried and calcined into charcoal, finely ground and applied externally, can be used to treat wounds after being mixed with sesame oil.

Olives

OLIVES CAN CLEAR THE lungs, moisturize the throat, generate fluids, relieve coughs, and detoxify. They are helpful for sore throat and throat redness caused by seasonal wind and fire. They can also prevent diphtheria and influenza. Fresh olive decoction can be used internally to treat acute bacterial dysentery.

Tofu

TOFU CAN CLEAR HEAT. It is more suitable for those with lung heat with yellow phlegm, sore throat, gastric heat with bad breath, and constipation. For individuals experiencing discomfort due to travel or changes in environment, such as itching all over the body or rash, eating tofu daily can help them adapt.

Overconsumption of tofu may cause abdominal distension and nausea, which can be alleviated by consuming turnips. Patients with carbuncles should avoid eating tofu.

Foods to Clear Heat and Detoxify

Green beans

THE COOLING EFFECT of green beans lies in the skin, while their detoxifying effect lies in the flesh. In folk medicine, consuming green bean soup or green bean soup with licorice is believed to have certain preventive and therapeutic effects against contact with toxic and harmful chemicals and gases. In traditional Chinese medicine, green beans are valued for their sweet and cold properties, and their ability to clear heat and detoxify, used in the treatment of carbuncles, swelling, and toxins. Green bean soup is a commonly prepared summer beverage at home, refreshing and appetizing, suitable for people of all ages.

Bitter gourd

ALTHOUGH BITTER IN taste, bitter gourd is cooling in nature. Fresh bitter gourd juice can be consumed or boiled into a soup for a stronger cooling effect. It can also be used as a supplementary food for those prone to internal heat accumulation. Bitter gourd is known for its ability to clear heat, improve vision, and detoxify.

Amaranth

AMARANTH CAN BE CONSUMED both as a vegetable and as medicine, with red amaranth being particularly medicinally potent. The seeds of amaranth contain a high concentration of lysine, which can complement the deficiency of amino acids found in grains. This is particularly significant for the growth and development of adolescents.

Pigweed is a type of amaranth. It can be consumed as a vegetable and is effective medicinally for acute enteritis, dysentery, pulmonary diseases, intestinal abscesses, breast abscesses, postpartum uterine bleeding, hemorrhoids bleeding, and edema associated with nephritis. In folk cuisine, pigweed is often mixed with minced meat as filling for dumplings and dumplings, which can help clear intestinal heat and stop diarrhea.

Cucumber

CUCUMBER CLEARS HEAT and quenches thirst, promotes diuresis, and detoxifies, which is helpful for edema in the limbs. It can be consumed raw or cooked; boiling with vinegar enhances its diuretic properties, while boiling with honey treats diarrhea. Acetic acid in fresh cucumber can inhibit the conversion of carbohydrates into fat, aiding in weight loss.

Cucumber juice can smooth wrinkles. Cucumber vines have a beneficial effect on lowering blood pressure and cholesterol. Cucumbers are cold in nature, and those with a cold stomach may experience abdominal pain if consumed excessively.

Elderly patients with chronic bronchitis should avoid eating cucumbers during exacerbations.

Foods for resolving phlegm, stopping coughing, and alleviating asthma

Sea cucumber

SEA CUCUMBER CAN DISSOLVE phlegm, soften hardness, soothe the liver, detoxify, stop coughing, lower blood pressure, nourish yin, and heal ulcers. It has therapeutic effects on acute and chronic bronchitis, pulmonary abscesses, bronchiectasis, and excessive phlegm with coughing.

Consuming sea cucumber to resolve phlegm does not damage the body's balance, nourishes yin and blood without retaining pathogenic factors. Externally, it has the ability to detoxify and reduce swelling. Coastal residents often use it for wet compresses on swollen lower limbs. It is effective in treating conditions such as yin deficiency with phlegm-heat and dry stools, as clinically proven.

Water chestnut

WATER CHESTNUT HAS the functions of clearing heat, resolving phlegm, eliminating accumulation, and promoting diuresis. It is suitable for conditions such as fever with thirst, constipation, lung dryness due to yin deficiency, phlegm-heat cough, and excessive liver yang.

Water chestnut shoots have diuretic and anti-edema effects, which can treat edema caused by nephritis. It is also suitable for those with a feeling of oppression in the chest.

Bamboo Shoots

BAMBOO SHOOTS HAVE been regarded as a delicacy among vegetables since ancient times. They possess the qualities of clearing heat and resolving phlegm, promoting urination and reducing swelling, as well as stopping diarrhea and dysentery. They are effective in treating phlegm-heat coughs, nephritis, or edema and ascites caused by heart disease or liver disease.

Drinking water boiled with fresh bamboo shoot roots as a tea substitute can lower blood cholesterol, aiding in weight loss and the treatment of hyperlipidemia and hypertension.

There are many types of bamboo shoots, including winter shoots harvested in winter, spring shoots harvested in spring, and whip shoots harvested in summer. Among these, winter shoots are of the highest quality, followed by spring shoots.

Luffa

Luffa is consumed when it is young and tender. It contains saponins, bitter substances, and a large amount of mucilage, as well as cucurbitine. The reticulated fiber left after peeling the mature luffa, known as loofah, can facilitate the flow of qi when burned. Luffa seeds can resolve phlegm and expel pus.

Pear

PEAR HAS THE FUNCTIONS of generating fluids, relieving thirst, moisturizing dryness, clearing heat, and resolving phlegm. Pear paste is mainly made from pear pulp, with added white sugar, egg whites, honey, and traditional Chinese medicine for resolving phlegm and stopping coughs. Regular consumption has significant therapeutic effects on chronic respiratory diseases. It is also suitable for those with dry mouth and tongue. Preparation method: Wash and core the pears, cut them into small pieces, and extract the juice through clean gauze; wash the fresh ginger, cut it into shreds, and extract the juice through clean gauze. Take the pear juice and simmer it over high heat, then reduce the heat and simmer until it thickens to a paste-like consistency. Add double the amount of honey and ginger juice, continue heating until boiling, then remove from heat and let it cool before bottling for later use. Take one tablespoon each time, dissolve it in boiling water, and drink it instead of tea several times a day. It is suitable for coughs with lung heat, yellow phlegm, and sore throat.

Nori Seaweed

NORI SEAWEED CAN DISSOLVE phlegm, clear heat, promote diuresis, and stop coughing. It is suitable for goiter, edema, gonorrhea, and athlete's foot. Residents in areas with endemic thyroid swelling often consume nori seaweed, which has a preventive and therapeutic effect. Additionally, nori seaweed can lower plasma cholesterol levels.

Mustard Greens

Fresh mustard greens are pungent and spicy. After being salt-pickled, they can be stir-fried and are often used in congee. Mustard greens seeds warm the middle, dispel cold, reduce swelling, and promote circulation. They induce sweating, disperse qi, and have a robust character. They can be consumed by those with colds without sweating, abdominal bloating and stagnation of qi, and phlegm obstruction.

Apricot Kernel

Sweet apricot kernels have a cough-suppressing and asthma-alleviating effect on patients with deficient lung qi and sudden asthma attacks. They do not possess bitter or adverse properties and can be used for chronic cough due to lung yin deficiency and deficient lung qi.

Luo Han Guo (Monk Fruit)

Luo Han Guo has cough-suppressing and heat-clearing properties, and it cools the blood and moistens the intestines. It is used to treat coughs, blood dryness, and heat-induced constipation.

Loquat

Loquat leaf preparations have the effects of reducing qi, resolving phlegm, clearing the lungs and stomach, and are used to treat coughs with lung heat, coughing up blood, nosebleeds, and heat-induced vomiting. However, they should not be taken by those with cold stomach vomiting and wind-cold coughs.

Foods for strengthening the spleen and resolving accumulation

Digestion-aiding Foods

WHITE RADISH WHITE radish can aid digestion, resolve phlegm, and soothe qi in the middle. It is helpful for indigestion, regurgitation, nosebleeds, abdominal distention due to food stagnation, and cough with excessive phlegm. There are many varieties of white radish, which can be eaten raw or cooked. It contains mustard oil and amylase, giving it a spicy taste that aids digestion and increases appetite.

Radishes also contain a certain amount of dietary fiber, which promotes gastrointestinal motility and bowel movements. It also has cough-suppressing and phlegm-resolving effects, providing some preventive effects against infectious diseases such as colds, meningitis, and diphtheria. Additionally, it can alleviate symptoms in patients suffering from coal gas poisoning.

Hawthorn

HAWTHORN AIDS IN DIGESTION, dissolves blood stasis, promotes diuresis, and stops diarrhea. It has vasodilating properties, lowers blood pressure, reduces cholesterol levels, and strengthens the heart. Hawthorn is often used for diarrhea due to indigestion and is effective in resolving meat accumulation.

It should be used cautiously in cases of weakness combined with food stagnation, often combined with herbs such as dang shen (Codonopsis) and bai zhu (Atractylodes) for optimal effect. It should be used with caution in cases of spleen deficiency and weak stomach without accumulation or stagnation, and excessive consumption of raw hawthorn can lead to noisy digestion and increased hunger.

Chicken Gizzard Membrane

CHICKEN GIZZARD MEMBRANE is an excellent product for nourishing the spleen and promoting health. It can invigorate the spleen and aid digestion, benefiting those with indigestion, abdominal distention, vomiting, regurgitation, diarrhea, and malnutrition in children. It is suitable for individuals with weak spleen and stomach constitutions, as well as children and those seeking to strengthen their bodies. It is also used for enuresis, nocturnal emission, gallstones, and urinary tract stones.

Malt

MALT IS MAINLY USED for conditions such as indigestion, especially in digesting wheat-based foods. The method is to take malt and chicken gizzard membrane, fry until yellow, grind into powder, mix with white sugar, and take with boiling water. Regular consumption can invigorate the spleen and stomach, aid digestion, and regulate liver qi.

It is suitable for individuals with weak spleen and stomach constitutions and liver depression. It can be cooked or fried and then ground into powder for consumption. Common health-preserving methods include malt porridge.

Excessive consumption can deplete vitality, induce miscarriage, and cause lactation cessation, so it is not suitable for individuals with weak qi, pregnant or lactating women.

Foods for nourishing the spleen and stomach

Pumpkin

PUMPKIN HAS THE EFFECTS of warming the middle and relieving asthma, as well as killing parasites and detoxifying. It is helpful for severe winter asthma and lung abscess when cooked into porridge.

Mature pumpkins contain starch, calcium, iron, and carotene. Young pumpkins are rich in vitamin C and glucose. There are many varieties of pumpkins with different names in various regions, but their functions are similar. In addition to expelling parasites, pumpkin seeds also have the effect of killing the larvae of blood flukes.

Jujube (Chinese Date)

JUJUBE NOURISHES THE spleen and stomach, replenishes qi and fluids, regulates the circulation of qi and blood, lowers blood lipid levels, and has anticancer properties. It also has the effects of inhibiting the central nervous system, protecting the liver, lowering cholesterol, and inhibiting the proliferation of cancer cells.

Jujube is mild in nature and can nourish the spleen and stomach, making it a commonly used food for regulating and supplementing the spleen and stomach. Jujube is sweet and warm; eating a small amount can invigorate the spleen, but eating too much can burden the spleen. It is not suitable for those with damp phlegm, accumulation, dental diseases, or parasitic diseases.

Chestnut

CHESTNUTS NOURISH THE stomach and invigorate the spleen, supplement the kidneys and strengthen the tendons, promote blood circulation and stop bleeding, and relieve coughing and dissolve phlegm. They primarily replenish kidney qi, making them suitable for kidney deficiencies, and are particularly effective in treating lower back and leg weakness.

However, they are not suitable for individuals with weak spleens and poor digestion, or those with excessive dampness and heat. They should not be consumed when there is an external pathogen invasion, or in cases of abdominal distention, malnutrition, malaria, dysentery, postpartum women, or young children.

Glutinous Rice

GLUTINOUS RICE SUPPLEMENTS the middle, boosts qi, strengthens the spleen, and stops diarrhea. It is effective for spleen deficiency diarrhea, excessive spontaneous sweating, and insufficient vitality. It can be cooked into porridge, used for making rice wine, or boiled into soup. However, when used for making cakes or pastries, its nature makes it difficult to digest, so it should be consumed sparingly.

The roots of glutinous rice, when brewed into a decoction, can relieve thirst and stop spontaneous sweating. Due to its sticky and difficult-to-digest nature, patients should avoid consuming it excessively.

Chinese Yam

CHINESE YAM NOURISHES the spleen, supplements the lungs, relieves thirst, and enriches the essence to consolidate the kidneys. It assists in the treatment of fatigue-induced coughing, excessive urination, and thirst.

Chinese yam has a sweet and neutral taste and enters the spleen, lungs, and kidneys. It nourishes without causing stagnation and is fragrant without being drying.

Chinese yam can be prepared as a dish, steamed after grinding into powder for making cakes, often used in sweet dishes. It can be sliced and boiled into a decoction for tea, or finely ground and cooked into porridge for consumption.

Foods for strengthening the spleen and resolving dampness

Coix Seed

COIX SEEDS HAVE THE functions of promoting diuresis, draining dampness, strengthening the spleen, and stopping diarrhea. Coix seeds have a mild and slightly cold nature, which doesn't harm the stomach and benefits the spleen without being greasy. Except for fried coix seeds used for treating diarrhea, other preparations typically use raw coix seeds.

Due to their rich nutritional content, coix seeds are often used for individuals with chronic illnesses and during the recovery period after an illness. They are considered beneficial medicinal foods for the elderly and children.

However, they should not be consumed by those with constipation, seminal emissions, pregnant women, insufficient semen, or excessive urination.

Broad Bean

BROAD BEANS ARE PRIMARILY used to treat edema. Broad bean leaves can treat pulmonary tuberculosis bleeding, gastrointestinal bleeding, and external bleeding.

Its flowers have the functions of cooling the blood and stopping bleeding, treating hemoptysis, bleeding, leukorrhea, and hypertension. Its stems can stop bleeding and diarrhea, treating various internal bleeding. Its husks have diuretic and dampness-draining effects, treating edema, athlete's foot, and difficulty in urination.

Eating too many mature broad beans can easily cause bloating, so they should be thoroughly cooked before consumption. In a few individuals, consuming broad beans may lead to acute hemolytic anemia.

Lima Bean

THERE ARE SEVERAL VARIETIES of lima beans, including white, black, and red-brown. White lima beans can be used as both food and medicine. They are effective in tonifying the spleen, regulating the middle, and resolving dampness. They can treat weakness of the spleen and stomach, resulting in poor appetite, vomiting, and diarrhea.

Black lima beans are used as food and not as medicine. Red lima beans are used as a liver-clearing medicine in folk medicine in Guangxi, treating the formation of cataracts in the eyes. Lima bean seeds, when used medicinally, tonify the spleen, clear heat, and resolve dampness. They can treat both acute and chronic diarrhea, as well as conditions such as leukorrhea. Lima bean leaves can be used to treat vomiting, diarrhea, sores, bruises, bleeding, hemorrhoids, and urinary tract infections.

Diuretic and Laxative Foods

Corn

CORN HELPS REGULATE the stomach and increase appetite, strengthening the spleen and stomach. It also has diuretic and stone-expelling properties, lowers cholesterol, blood pressure, and blood sugar levels. It is beneficial for conditions such as hypertension, hyperlipidemia, urinary tract stones, chronic nephritis, and diabetes.

For diuretic effects, corn silk is preferred, while corn oil is preferred for lowering cholesterol.

Red Adzuki Beans

RED ADZUKI BEANS HAVE the effects of diuresis, dampness removal, reducing swelling, and detoxification. They are effective in treating ascites, spleen deficiency with water swelling, and recurrent edema. They are often used to make red bean soup, red bean porridge, or ground into a fine powder for use as a filling.

In traditional medicine, red bean soup is used to nourish the blood, often cooked with red dates and longan fruit. Red adzuki bean leaves, flowers, and sprouts are also used as medicine. The leaves can stop frequent urination. The flowers are used to treat dysentery, alcohol-induced headaches, carbuncles, and erysipelas. The sprouts are used to treat rectal bleeding and miscarriage with leakage of the fetus.

Winter Melon

WINTER MELON HAS LOW sugar content and high water content. It has diuretic properties, reducing swelling and eliminating excess body fat accumulation. It has beneficial effects for patients with diabetes, coronary heart disease, arteriosclerosis, hypertension, and obesity.

Winter melon has low sodium content, making it an ideal vegetable for patients with kidney disease and edema. It has a cooling nature. Those who are weak and cold or have chronic diarrhea should avoid consuming it.

Lettuce Stem

THERE ARE MANY VARIETIES of lettuce stems, including white lettuce stem, pointed lettuce stem, as well as purple and flower leaf lettuce stems. There are also various methods of consumption, including cold mixing, stir-frying, sun-drying with salt pickling, and fermentation. It is effective for early-stage mastitis.

Fresh leaves boiled into a decoction can promote bowel movements and treat edema.

Carp Fish

PEOPLE OFTEN EAT FISH for improving eyesight. The scales of carp are formed from the dermis of the skin and are composed of transformed collagen known as fish scale keratin. They function in dispersing and stopping bleeding, used to treat vomiting blood, bleeding, irregular menstruation with excessive flow, abdominal pain due to blood stasis, hemorrhoids, and fish bone stuck in the throat.

Carp can promote diuresis, reduce swelling, expel gas, promote lactation, alleviate coughing, stabilize pregnancy, reduce jaundice, and calm agitation.

Crucian Carp

CRUCIAN CARP STRENGTHENS the spleen and stomach, alleviates thirst, and resolves small intestinal hernia. It is helpful for individuals with cold spleen and stomach, poor appetite, weakness, and lack of strength.

If crucian carp soup is given to postpartum women to induce lactation, it is advisable to cook it with water until the fish soup becomes slightly thick and milky white in color.

The burnt ashes of its bones, when applied externally, can treat yellow vesicles and abscesses.

Spinach

SPINACH CLEARS HEAT, relieves irritability, quenches thirst, and promotes bowel movements. It is used to treat urinary obstruction, intestinal and stomach heat accumulation, chest stuffiness, constipation, and nyctalopia. It is not suitable for those with weak constitution and loose stools. Patients with nephritis and kidney stones should not consume it.

Honey

HONEY SUPPLEMENTS THE middle burner, moisturizes dryness, alleviates urgency, detoxifies, lowers blood pressure, and promotes bowel movements.

Honey can enhance the body's resistance, energize the body, regulate the spleen and stomach functions, and treat gastritis, constipation, gastric and duodenal ulcers. It also has the ability to promote tissue regeneration and accelerate wound healing. Additionally, it is beneficial for nourishing the myocardium in patients with heart disease and has therapeutic effects on individuals with neurasthenia and hepatitis.

Due to differences in the source of bees and nectar, honey can be categorized into white honey and yellow honey, with honey from fruit flowers being the best choice due to its sweet and pure qualities.

Foods to promote blood circulation

Canola

CANOLA PROMOTES BLOOD circulation, dispels stasis, reduces swelling, and detoxifies. It is effective for conditions such as hemorrhage due to overexertion, persistent bloody dysentery, abdominal pain, restlessness of the mind, and various unidentified swellings and toxins.

In early spring, the tender shoots of fresh vegetables are delicious when stir-fried. Later, after being picked and dried, they can be salted and chopped into jars, known as pickled yellow vegetables, which taste even better.

Both fresh vegetables and pickled vegetables have the effect of clearing heat and detoxifying. Patients with measles, skin ulcers, and eye diseases should not consume it.

Judas's Ear Mushroom

JUDAS'S EAR MUSHROOM moisturizes the lungs, stops coughing, promotes urination, and invigorates blood circulation. It is effective for lung deficiency coughing up blood, postpartum blood stasis, and retention of the placenta.

The skin of Judas's ear mushroom is brownish and has a slightly astringent and numbing taste. It is generally peeled before cooking and consumption.

When mashed and mixed with ginger juice, it can be applied externally to treat various unidentified swellings and painful inflammations.

Peach

FRESH PEACHES NOURISH the body fluids, moisten the intestines, invigorate blood circulation, relieve asthma, and lower blood pressure. They are suitable for quenching thirst in summer, relieving menstrual pain, treating amenorrhea, and alleviating constipation in the elderly. This fruit contains a high amount of potassium, making it suitable for patients with edema as an adjunct food when taking diuretics. Peaches are commonly eaten fresh or preserved.

Due to their mild blood circulation-promoting and blood-stasis-resolving effects, they are recommended for consumption by women during menstruation.

Adolescent girls often experience irregular menstruation in the period after menarche, and eating more peaches or preserved peaches is especially beneficial for those experiencing menstrual pain due to excessive consumption of cold food.

Crab

CRAB HAS THE EFFECTS of nourishing yin, replenishing marrow, clearing heat, and dispersing blood stasis. It is effective for fractures, tendon injuries, postpartum occipital pain in women, and can be consumed with hot alcohol for good effect.

Crab is a delicacy in autumn and can be cooked in various ways such as steaming, salting, marinating, or soaking in wine, but it should be washed thoroughly and fully cooked. As it has a salty and cold nature, it should not be consumed together with persimmons. It is often dipped in ginger vinegar sauce, which not only enhances the flavor but also reduces its coldness.

In case of crab poisoning, drinking a decoction of perilla leaves and fresh ginger or ingesting ginger juice can be effective.

Vinegar

VINEGAR PROMOTES BLOOD circulation, disperses blood stasis, aids digestion, dissolves accumulations, reduces swelling, softens indurations, and detoxifies wounds. As a condiment, vinegar not only enhances flavor but also increases gastric acid secretion, stimulates appetite, aids digestion, and has some antimicrobial properties.

In case of overconsumption of fishy food or accumulation of cold and raw vegetables and fruits, crushed fresh ginger mixed with rice vinegar can be consumed.

It is not advisable for individuals with excessive dampness in the spleen and stomach, paralysis, muscle spasms, or those experiencing the early stages of external pathogens to consume vinegar. Healthy individuals should also avoid excessive consumption. When cooking with vinegar, copper utensils should be avoided as vinegar can dissolve copper, leading to copper poisoning.

Wine

WINE IS ONE OF THE oldest medicines in the world, with aged wine considered superior. Medicinal wines are often made by soaking various types of single or compound Chinese medicinal herbs in liquor, typically using distilled spirits, to enhance the medicinal properties due to the warmth and dispersing nature of alcohol, allowing the medicinal effects to quickly reach the entire body through the meridians.

Wine is also commonly used as a seasoning in cooking to eliminate odors.

Foods to stop bleeding

Watercress

FRESH WATERCRESS CLEARS heat, cools blood, and detoxifies. Watercress can be used to make soup, boiled with noodles, stir-fried, blanched with boiling water and served cold, or used for pickling. When cooked with pork, it can give the meat a purple color and tender texture.

Watercress can be consumed raw or cooked, and it is suitable for both vegetarian and non-vegetarian diets. It possesses various therapeutic effects.

Purple watercress contains insulin-like components. Regular consumption can improve appetite, making it particularly suitable for diabetes patients. It can also clear heat from the stomach and intestines, moisten the intestines, and promote bowel movements, making it suitable for bad breath and constipation.

Burdock

BURDOCK ROOTS AND LEAVES, after drying, are used in medicine. It has the functions of clearing heat, reducing inflammation, stopping bleeding, restoring liver function, and promoting liver cell regeneration. Therefore, it can be used as a vegetable for those with hepatitis, hematuria, and other liver and urinary tract diseases, and regular consumption is recommended.

Daylily

DAYLILY NOURISHES BLOOD and stops bleeding. It is preferable to consume processed dried daylily rather than fresh or spoiled ones to avoid poisoning. It should not be stir-fried alone. After soaking and cleaning, it is appropriate to cook it thoroughly by stir-frying or stewing. It has the function of nourishing blood and replenishing deficiency. Stewed with meat, it can nourish the body, promote lactation, treat anemia, and calm fetal restlessness.

Regular consumption can also clear heat, relieve irritability, and promote peaceful sleep for those who are restless and sleep poorly due to emotional distress.

Commonly used foods for tonifying qi

MEDICINAL FOODS SUCH as ginseng, deer antler, and Cordyceps, when used alone, have tonifying effects. Medicinal porridge is made by cooking common tonifying foods or medicinal herbs together with rice, and it also has the advantage of combining food with medicine. Tonifying medicinal cuisine is prepared by cooking medicinal herbs with food simultaneously. Not only does it have the combined effects of food and medicine, but it is also popular because of its exquisite preparation and delightful taste, aroma, and appearance.

Potato

POTATOES ARE EFFECTIVE in tonifying qi, strengthening the spleen, and regulating the middle burner. They are helpful for post-illness spleen and stomach deficiency with cold, shortness of breath, fatigue, as well as for gastric and duodenal ulcer pain, and habitual constipation.

Potato juice can be used to treat scalds, and applying vinegar externally can treat parotitis.

Due to the presence of solanine in potato sprouts and skins, it can destroy red blood cells. Severe poisoning can lead to cerebral congestion, edema, inflammation of the gastrointestinal mucosa, and conjunctivitis.

If potatoes sprout, they should be deeply dug and the skin near the sprout should be peeled off. Then soak them in water and cook for a long time to remove and destroy solanine, preventing poisoning from excessive consumption. People with spleen and stomach deficiency with cold tendency and susceptibility to diarrhea should eat less.

Fragrant Mushroom

FRAGRANT MUSHROOM HAS a pleasant aroma and delicious taste, which can stimulate the appetite and reduce blood lipid levels. It is particularly suitable for patients with hyperlipidemia and can also be used as a food for children with rickets to assist in treatment. The polysaccharides in fragrant mushrooms have certain immunomodulatory and anticancer effects, which are beneficial for patients with tumors.

Fragrant mushrooms contain compounds such as eritadenine that can lower blood lipid levels. Additionally, they are rich in calcium and phosphorus, making them a natural food for preventing rickets.

Wild fragrant mushrooms should be avoided after heatstroke, childbirth, or illness, as they can be easily confused with poisonous mushrooms. Ingesting them by mistake can lead to poisoning, and severe cases can be fatal.

Loach

LOACH TONIFIES THE middle burner, dispels dampness, clears heat, and strengthens yang. It is a good food for treating liver disease, gallbladder disease, diabetes, and urinary system diseases. It has a choleretic effect.

Loach tonifies while also having a clearing effect, making it suitable for various illnesses.

Osmanthus Fish

OSMANTHUS FISH TONIFIES qi and blood, benefits the spleen and stomach, and helps dissolve bone spurs. It is an essential food therapy for those with deficiency fatigue, and it is recommended for patients with pulmonary tuberculosis. Individuals suffering from cold and damp conditions should avoid consuming it.

Japonica Rice

JAPONICA RICE PORRIDGE is a staple food for residents of Southeast Asia and other regions, serving as the main source of energy for the body. It can tonify the middle burner, strengthen the spleen and stomach, and alleviate irritability and thirst.

Japonica rice is nutritionally rich, with most nutrients found in the bran. Therefore, it is not advisable to consume refined grains excessively to prevent the loss of minerals and vitamins due to the removal of bran.

Japonica rice contains starch, protein, vitamins, and other substances. Its phosphorus content is slightly higher than that of glutinous rice, while its amylose content is slightly lower than that of glutinous rice.

Rice and Wheat

WHEAT GERM CONTAINS abundant vitamin E, which can combat aging and prevent senility, making it suitable for consumption by the elderly. Floating wheat is sweet and cold in nature, possessing the effects of calming nerves, stopping night sweats, alleviating dry mouth and tongue, nourishing body fluids, and nourishing the heart qi. It is commonly used to treat conditions such as deficiency heat with excessive cold, night sweats, dry mouth, restlessness, and insomnia.

Chicken

CHICKEN MEAT IS RICH in protein and contains unsaturated fatty acids in its fat, making it a preferable protein source for the elderly and patients with cardiovascular diseases. It is particularly suitable as a nourishing food for individuals with weak constitution, recovering from illness, or postpartum, especially when consumed as chicken meat or chicken soup, with black-bone chicken being the preferred choice.

It can be used for conditions such as deficiency fatigue, bone-steaming heat, spleen deficiency with diarrhea, diabetes mellitus, uterine bleeding, leukorrhea, and spermatorrhea.

Chicken wings and chicken feet are known to exacerbate wind, generate phlegm, and aggravate internal heat, so they should be avoided by individuals with hyperactivity of liver yang. Those with unresolved excess conditions or lingering pathogenic factors should also refrain from consumption.

Quail

QUAIL IS CONSIDERED a beneficial nourishing food due to its delicious taste, easy digestibility, and high nutritional value. It is suitable for consumption by pregnant women, lactating mothers, and the elderly or individuals with weakened constitution. Additionally, it serves as a good dietary option for patients with hyperlipidemia, hypertension, coronary heart disease, and obesity.

Quail has the ability to tonify the spleen, resolve accumulation, nourish the liver and kidneys, and strengthen tendons and bones. It is particularly suitable for individuals with liver and kidney yin deficiency or those experiencing soreness and weakness in the lower back and knees.

Common Blood-Nourishing Foods

Carrot

CARROT IS A RARE COMBINATION of fruit, vegetable, and medicinal properties. Beta-carotene in carrots can be quickly converted into vitamin A in the human body, maintaining the health of eyes and skin, preventing respiratory infections, and regulating metabolism. Since vitamin A is fat-soluble, consuming carrots raw in salads is not conducive to absorption; it is more effective to stir-fry them with oil or cook them with meat.

Carrots can lower blood pressure, reduce blood sugar, and strengthen the heart, making them suitable dietary therapy for patients with coronary heart disease and diabetes. For people who smoke regularly, drinking half a cup of carrot juice daily can help protect the lungs.

Grapes

GRAPES ARE EFFECTIVE in nourishing qi and blood, strengthening tendons and bones, facilitating urination, securing pregnancy, and alleviating irritability and thirst. However, consuming them in excess can cause restlessness and dim vision. This food is suitable for individuals with gallbladder inflammation, gallstones, and those with a reduced white blood cell count.

After drying, grapes have an increased content of sugar and iron, making them an excellent tonic for children, women, and those who are weak or anemic.

Longan Fruit

LONGAN FRUIT CAN TONIFY the heart and spleen, nourish qi and blood, calm the mind, strengthen the spleen to stop diarrhea, and promote diuresis to reduce swelling. It is beneficial for individuals with spleen deficiency leading to diarrhea, postpartum edema in women, spleen deficiency due to overexertion, and restlessness with insomnia.

Longan fruit is rich in sugars, which are easily digested and absorbed monosaccharides. It is also high in iron and rich in vitamin B2, which can alleviate uterine contractions and sagging, playing a role in maintaining pregnancy.

Lychee

FRESH LYCHEE PULP IS sweet and juicy, quenching thirst and considered a premium fruit. Lychee can nourish yin and blood, strengthen the spleen to stop diarrhea, warm the middle burner, regulate qi, and descend rebellious qi. It is helpful for individuals with long-standing spleen deficiency leading to diarrhea, elderly individuals experiencing nighttime diarrhea, incessant hiccups, women with weak constitution and anemia, and those with deficient qi and cold stomach.

Individuals with yin deficiency and excessive internal heat should use caution when consuming lychees.

Peanuts

PEANUTS HAVE A SWEET and mild nature, with therapeutic effects such as tonifying the body, nourishing the spleen and stomach, moistening the lungs and resolving phlegm, regulating qi and nourishing blood, promoting diuresis and reducing swelling, and stopping bleeding and promoting lactation.

Peanuts are high in oil content and rich in protein, and they are easily digested and absorbed by the body. Modern studies have reported that peanuts can lower cholesterol, prevent skin aging, and enhance memory, making them a longevity food.

A stew made with peanuts and pig lungs, seasoned lightly and consumed together with the soup, can treat chronic coughs and whooping cough in children. Stewing peanuts with lily bulbs and American ginseng, and then adding honey for consumption, has a good effect in treating dry cough due to lung yin deficiency and hoarseness. People with cold and damp conditions or those experiencing slippery stools should avoid consumption.

Moldy peanuts have carcinogenic effects and should not be consumed. Peanut husks have a sweet and slightly astringent nature, with excellent hemostatic effects. They are used for various internal and external bleeding conditions, including hemophilia, idiopathic thrombocytopenic purpura, functional uterine bleeding, liver disease bleeding, and trauma-related bleeding. After administration, they can quickly stop bleeding and accelerate the resolution of hematomas.

Beef

BEEF CAN STRENGTHEN the spleen, invigorate the stomach, and replenish qi and blood, with extremely high nutritional value. It is suitable for individuals with chronic illness and weakness, qi deficiency leading to sinking, shortness of breath, sallow complexion, diarrhea, and cold extremities, who can consume beef stewed in soup. For postoperative patients, beef can be combined with red dates to tonify the middle burner, nourish qi, assist muscle growth, and promote healing.

It should be avoided in cases of excessive internal heat.

Foods to assist the yang energy

Walnut

WALNUT KERNELS ARE essential for nourishing the liver and kidneys, and strengthening the tendons and bones, making them effective in treating backaches, leg pains, and all kinds of musculoskeletal pain. They can also strengthen teeth and blacken hair, treat asthenia with panting and coughing, deficiency of qi not returning to its source, deficiency-cold in the lower burner, frequent urination, urinary tract stones, and various gynecological disorders.

Walnut kernels have a moistening and nourishing quality, suitable for the elderly with deficiency patterns and constipation due to post-illness fluid deficiency, as well as symptoms such as dizziness and tinnitus.

Chinese Chives

CHINESE CHIVES HAVE a warming and yang-tonifying effect, promote qi circulation, alleviate pain and numbness, promote blood circulation, and lower blood lipid levels. They are helpful for acute chest pain and various blood disorders. Chinese chives are beneficial for individuals with high blood lipid levels and coronary heart disease.

In addition to the role of fiber, volatile essential oils, and sulfur compounds in Chinese chives also have lipid-lowering effects. Chinese chives have an excitatory effect on the isolated uterus; they also have inhibitory effects on dysentery, typhoid fever, Escherichia coli, and Staphylococcus aureus.

Lamb

LAMB IS CONSIDERED warm and sweet in nature and has long been regarded as a tonic for yang, particularly suitable for consumption in winter. It provides more calories than beef, and eating lamb in winter can promote blood circulation to keep warm. Therefore, it is beneficial for the elderly, the weak, and those with deficient yang who experience cold hands and feet.

Angelica Lamb Soup: Wash the lamb, and add angelica, astragalus, codonopsis, spring onion, ginger, salt, and cooking wine into a pot with an appropriate amount of water. Bring to a boil over high heat, then simmer over low heat until the lamb is tender. Season with a moderate amount of MSG before serving. This soup is suitable for individuals with blood deficiency, as well as those who are weak after illness or childbirth, experience cold and painful sensations in the abdomen, suffer from uterine bleeding due to blood deficiency and cold, or have various types of anemia.

Sheep Milk

COMPARED TO COW'S MILK, goat's milk is richer in fat and protein, while sheep's milk has even higher levels of fat and protein. Historically, great importance was placed on the tonic properties of sheep's milk, which was considered an excellent remedy for nourishing the lungs, moistening dryness, and stopping coughs. It was believed to be effective in treating lung cancer, hemoptysis, and other conditions.

Foods to nourish the yin

Silver Ear Fungus

SILVER EAR FUNGUS IS beneficial for lung yin deficiency, cough due to deficiency, phlegm tinged with blood, and thirst due to yin deficiency. Silver ear fungus is a type of edible fungus and a nutritious tonic. It is also a medicinal ingredient for strengthening the body. It can be consumed regularly by individuals with high blood pressure, arteriosclerosis, constipation, and excessive menstruation. The polysaccharides in silver ear fungus can enhance the body's immune system, stimulate lymphocytes, strengthen the phagocytic capacity of white blood cells, and excite bone marrow hematopoietic function. Polysaccharide A also has certain anti-radiation effects.

Chinese Cabbage

CHINESE CABBAGE HAS the effects of clearing heat, relieving irritability, promoting digestion, and diuresis. Chinese cabbage is sweet, mild, and neutral in nature. When cooked with meat, it enhances the taste, nourishes the stomach, and has relatively mild therapeutic effects. Long-term consumption does not result in significant side effects.

Milk

MILK IS RICH IN NUTRIENTS, containing not only fats, proteins, carbohydrates, and vitamins but also pantothenic acid, inositol, and whey acid. The cholesterol content in milk fat is lower than that in meat and eggs, making it a very suitable nutritional food for the elderly.

Chicken eggs

EGGS ARE A WELL-KNOWN nutritious food, containing complete proteins. The proteins mainly consist of albumin and globulin, which are essential for infant growth and have a high absorption rate due to their similarity to human protein composition. Eggs also contain a variety of minerals, with iron content being richer than that in milk, making them an ideal food for the elderly, children, pregnant and lactating women, as well as patients with weak health.

Eggs nourish yin and moisturize dryness, nourish the heart, and calm the mind. Egg whites clear the lungs and promote throat health, while also clearing heat and detoxifying. Egg yolks nourish yin, nourish blood, moisturize dryness, extinguish wind, and invigorate the spleen and stomach.

Turtle

TURTLE MEAT NOURISHES yin, tonifies deficiency, stops diarrhea, and treats malaria. While turtles and tortoises are often mentioned together, the latter mainly focuses on nourishing yin, replenishing blood, stopping bleeding, and strengthening bones, whereas turtle meat is better known for its ability to clear deficiency heat and remove blood stasis. Turtle blood is used to treat bone tuberculosis. The plastron of turtles, known as turtle shell, is an important medicine for nourishing yin, tonifying the kidneys, nourishing blood, and replenishing the heart.

Turtle meat has been found to inhibit tumor cells and enhance immune function. It is suitable for those suffering from pulmonary tuberculosis, bloody stools, hemoptysis, hemorrhoids, frequent fever in the hands and feet, leg weakness, chronic nephritis, hepatitis, and other conditions.

Duck

DUCK MEAT NOURISHES yin, nurtures the stomach, promotes diuresis, reduces swelling, strengthens the spleen, and tonifies deficiency. Difference between chicken and duck meat: Chicken is suitable for people with symptoms of cold intolerance and weakness, such as general debility, emaciation, weak digestion with little appetite, diarrhea, edema, pale menstrual blood, thin vaginal discharge, insufficient lactation after childbirth, post-illness weakness, fatigue, and impotence.

Duck meat, on the other hand, is suitable for people with heat or fire in the body, especially those with low-grade fever, weakness, dry stools, edema, night sweats, spermatorrhea, scanty menstruation in women, dry throat, and thirst.

For more information about Traditional Chinese Medicine, please visit www.tcmhealthylife.com.